Evoke Embrace Evolve

A 33-day journey to manifesting your heart and mind's desire

Published by:
Liza Boubari, C.C.Ht, C.S.Mc
www.HealWithin.com

ISBN #978-1-7333126-3-9

May the pages in this 33-day calendar find words that grow the desire in you to improve your personal life, relationships, and your overall wellness by tapping within yourSELF.

With heartfelt dedication to all the brave women making way through these interesting times, called life.

May you Evoke what was, Embrace what is and Evolve to what will be – because You Matter

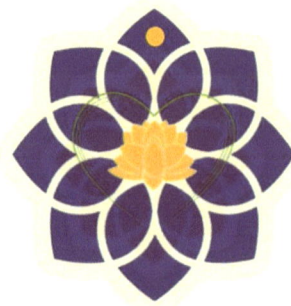

ME TIME

Evoke Embrace Evolve

A 33-day journey to manifesting your heart and mind's desire.

If you dedicated 15 to 20 minutes a day all to yourself, what will you discover? You'll discover your personal pattern and ready to Step Into the Best You!

Why You Need This - Now more than ever?! Through this 33 Calendar/Journal, you are guided to take an honest look at your life and explore what it truly takes to shift thoughts and habits, and design extraordinary dimensions of you!

Instructions:
- Sit back, relax and imagine what you want for yourself on the most important journey in your life.
- Set aside time to only read the date and page of the day.
- Fill out your journey and answers for each date on the blank pages provided.

It is best if you do this first thing in the morning or just before you go to sleep each night. This way your subconscious will recall what you want in life with new positive shifts and habits.

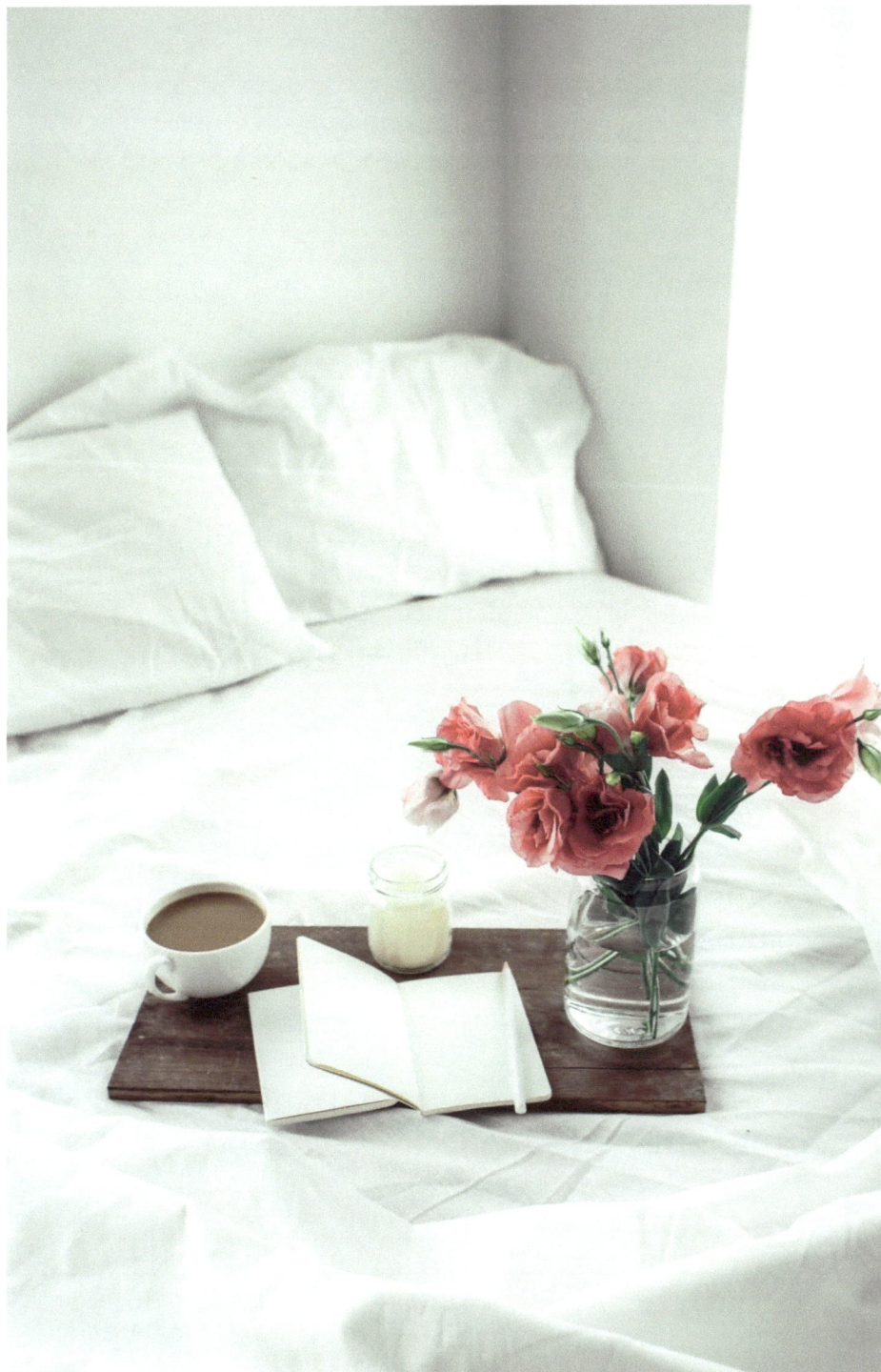

Why 33 days?
Liza's 33 Days New Habit Forming Theory

You may have heard the phrase "It takes 21 days to form a habit."

Liza's philosophy is that it takes '33 consecutive days of repeating the same thing over and over – either good or bad, to change and form a new habit.
Are you wondering why 33 days instead of 21 days?

We as humans are creatures of habit and function in a society where everything is measured by "time." This means - we know and understand seconds, minutes, hours, days, weeks, and months. The most days in a month are 31. So if we continue a new routine for over 33 consecutive days, then we have done it for over an entire month and are already into the next month. Follow me so far?

Most think and feel "If I can do it for over a month, I wonder if I can continue it for the next 33 days," thus placing the new programming into action for the next month.

Simply put; instead of coming short in the month (21 days), you have now accomplished something you did not believe imaginable. While your entire thought process was to do something for 33 days continually, the pressure and the discomfort of "possible failure" is lifted ... and by the second month, your subconscious is already forming the new habit. Bingo!

You now create a new pattern of thoughts and conquer old habits. Saying to yourself: "I can do this" - "it works"! Success feeds success! And what is "it"? IT is YOU.

DEAR FUTURE,

I'M READY

Show Up, Stand Up & Speak Up

I MATTER

Day 1

What are your feelings right now? Write till you shift from thinking to feeling.

- If my life were a movie, what would the overall message be - what is my story?
- What gets me excited and motivated?
- What do I stand for, feel, passionate about, or deeply believe in?

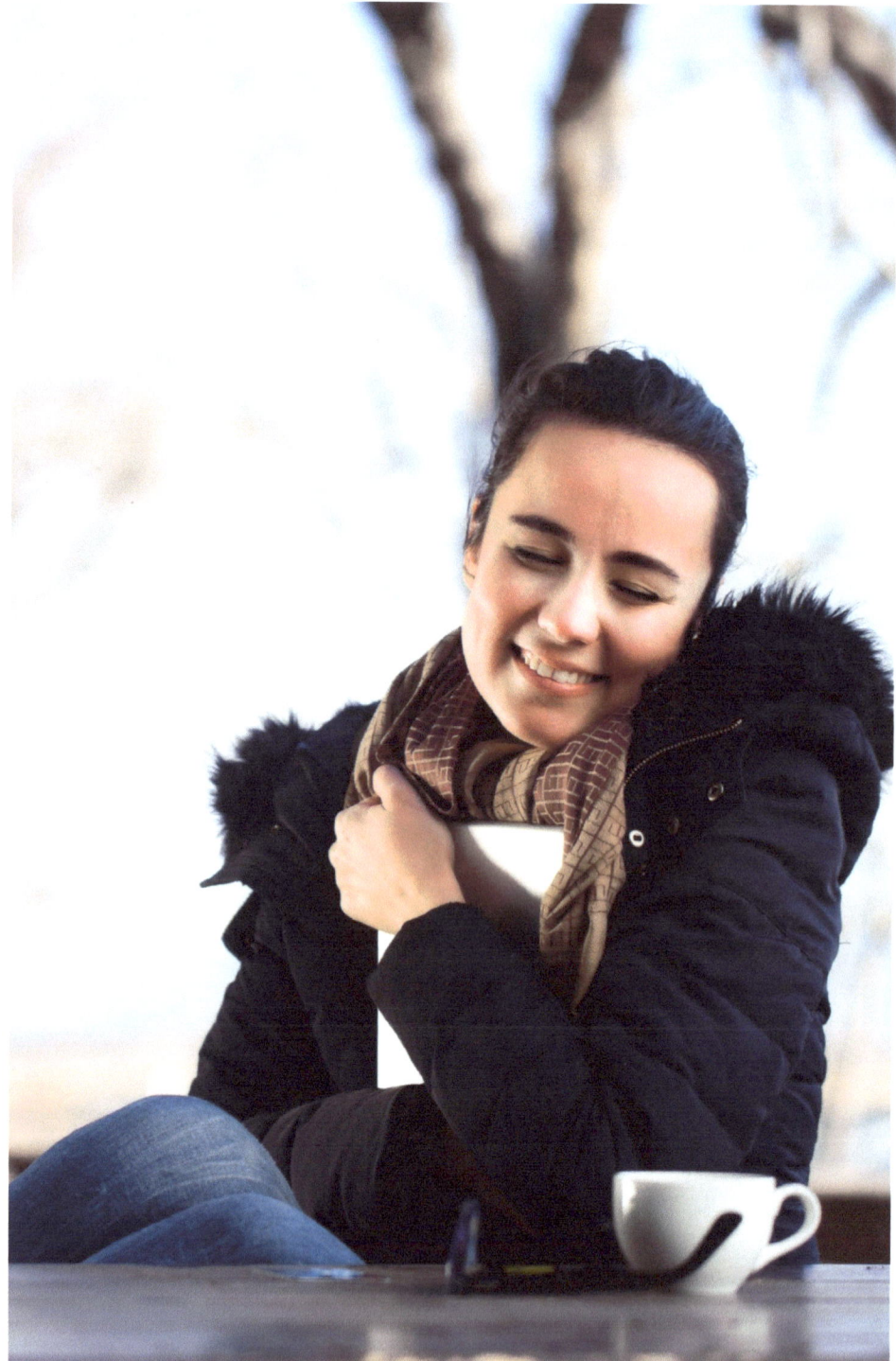

Day 2

Everything in life stems from self-esteem.

- What is my struggle through my journey that is bigger than me?
- What is something I am willing to fight for or love?
- What gives me reason to wake up each day?

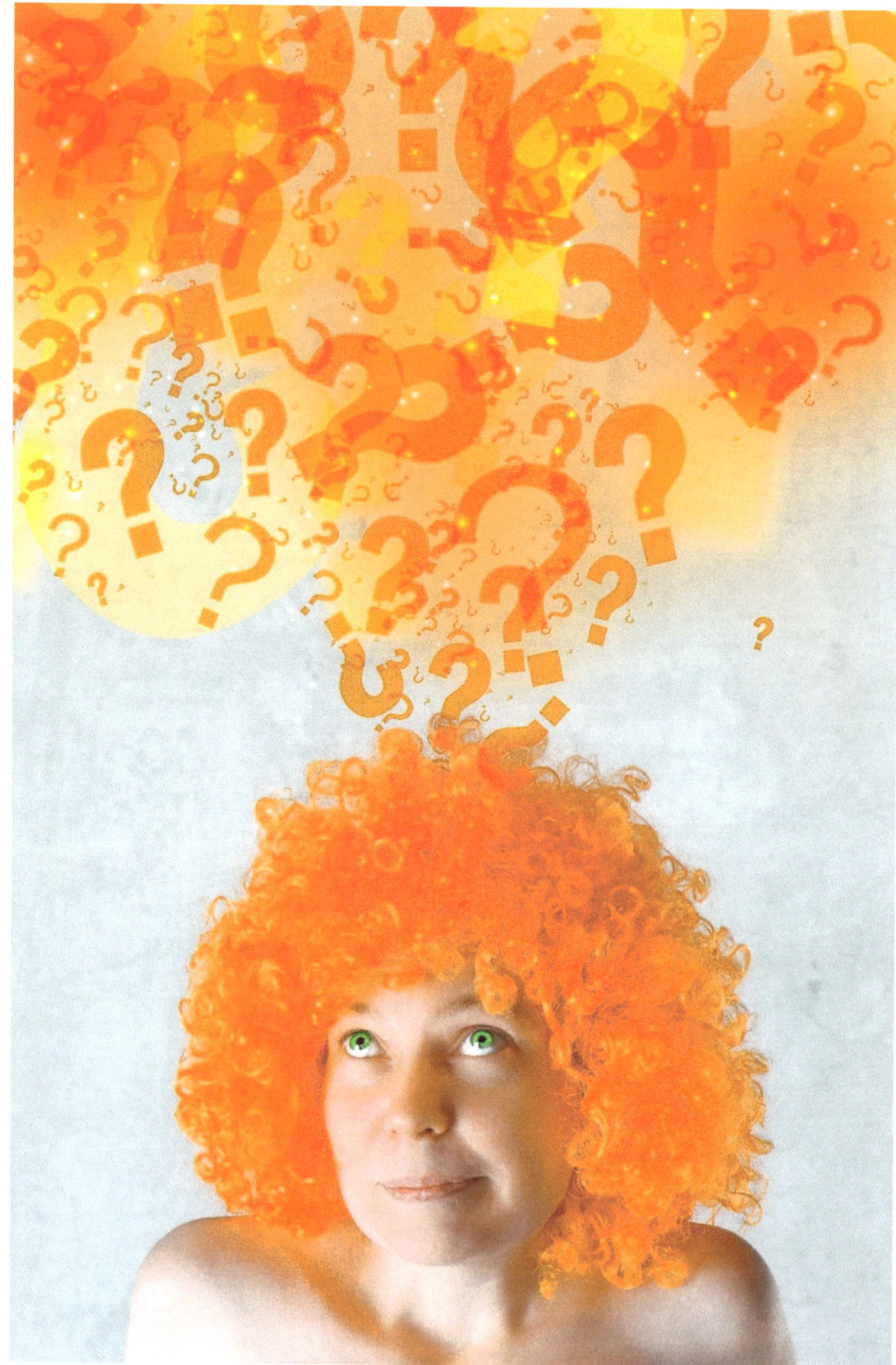

Day 3

Why is this YOUR passion?

What is my driving force or passion?
- Is it a book?
- Is it a cause?
- Is it a course?
- Is it a lifestyle?
- Is it my family?
- Is it a business?

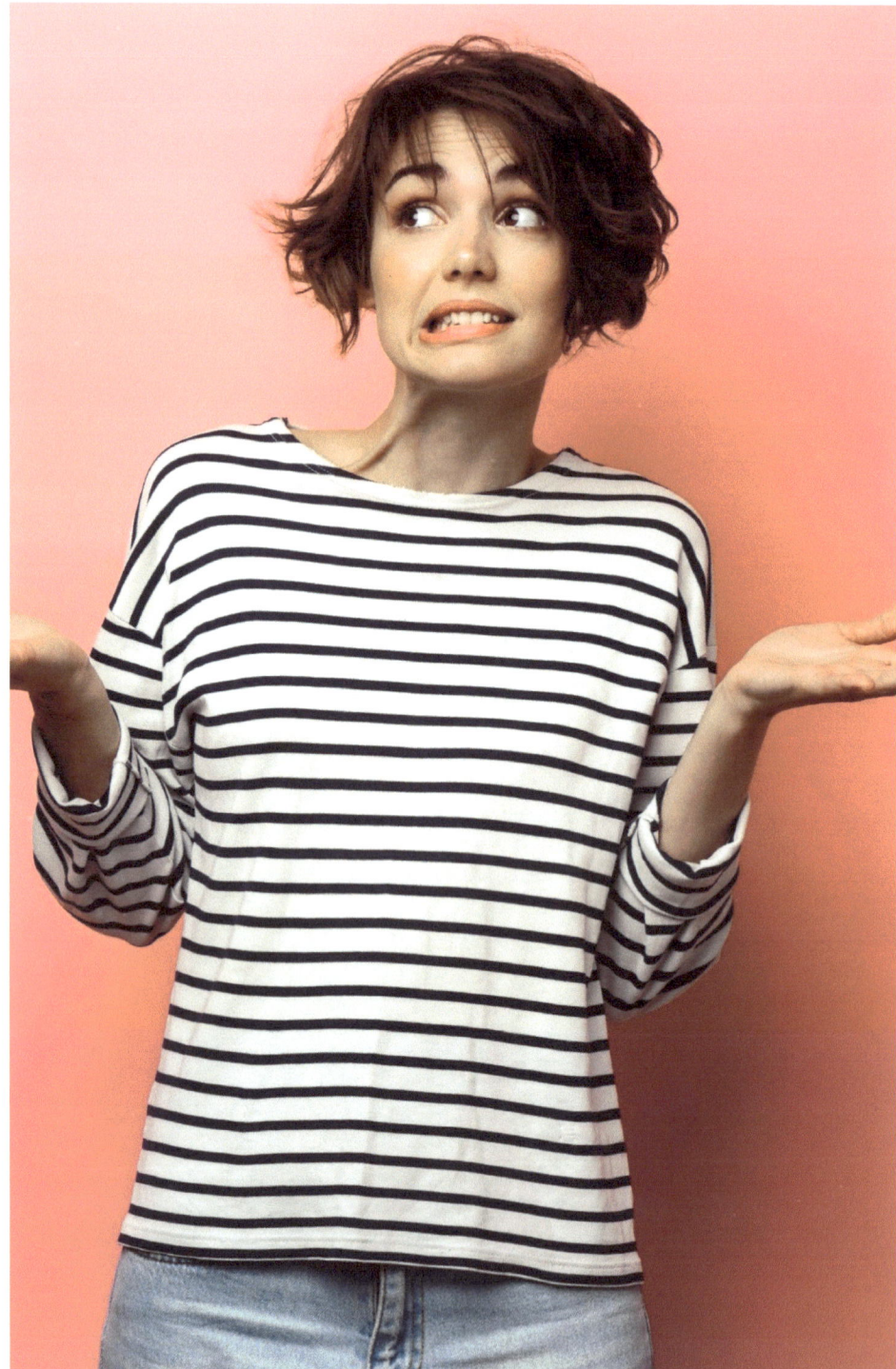

Day 4

What daily rituals do you have?
(for example)

- Wake up early
- Meditate
- Walk - Exercise
- Eat a healthy breakfast
- Write in a journal
- Call a loved one

How do these rituals help me feel better and more productive through my day?

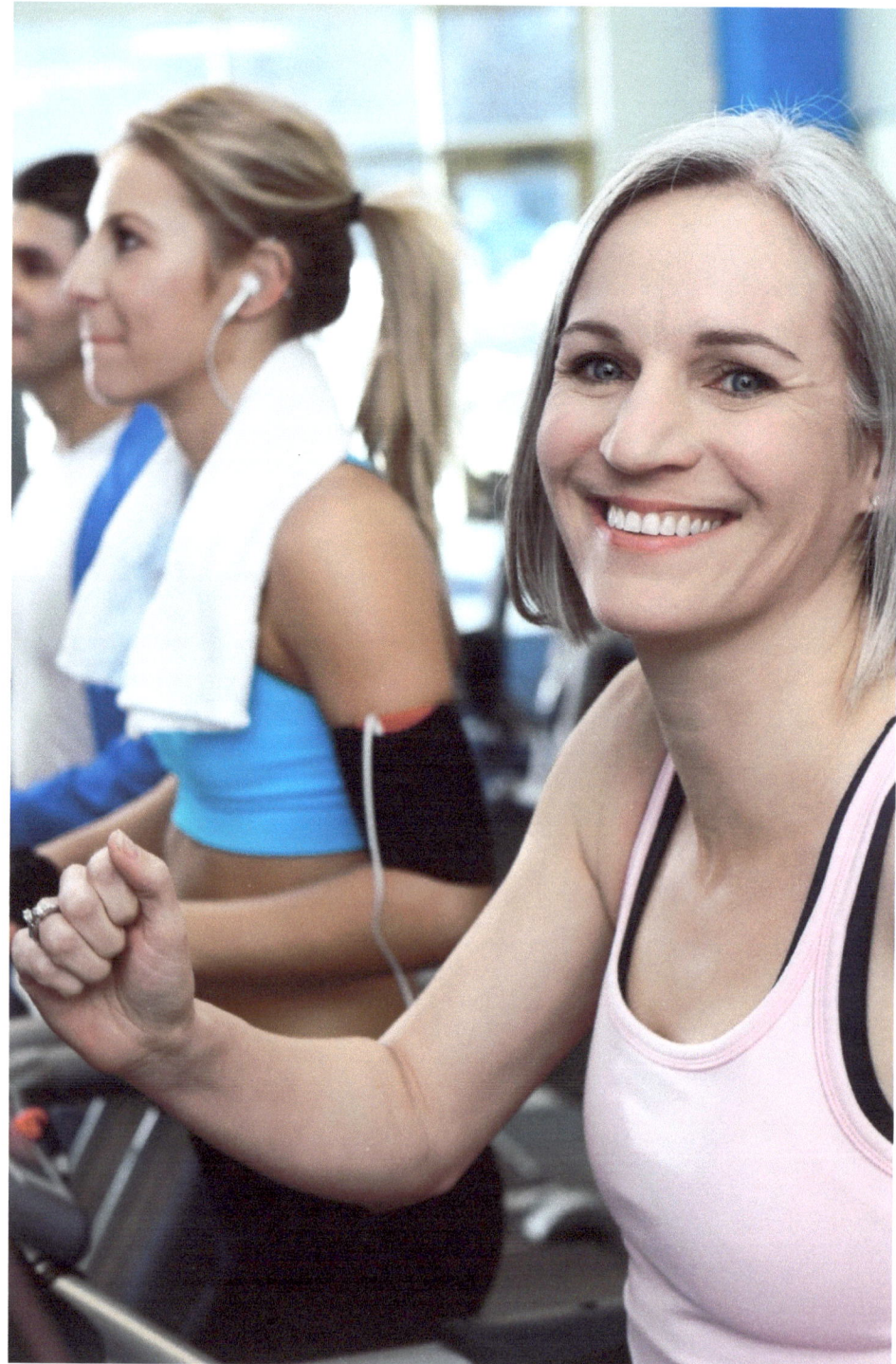

Day 5

Think of a habit or behavior you want to change.

Most of us don't make a change until it really hurts us, or the rewards are far greater.

- What 3 words define the best of who I am?
- What is great about my life?
- What is my BIG why right now – what excites me?

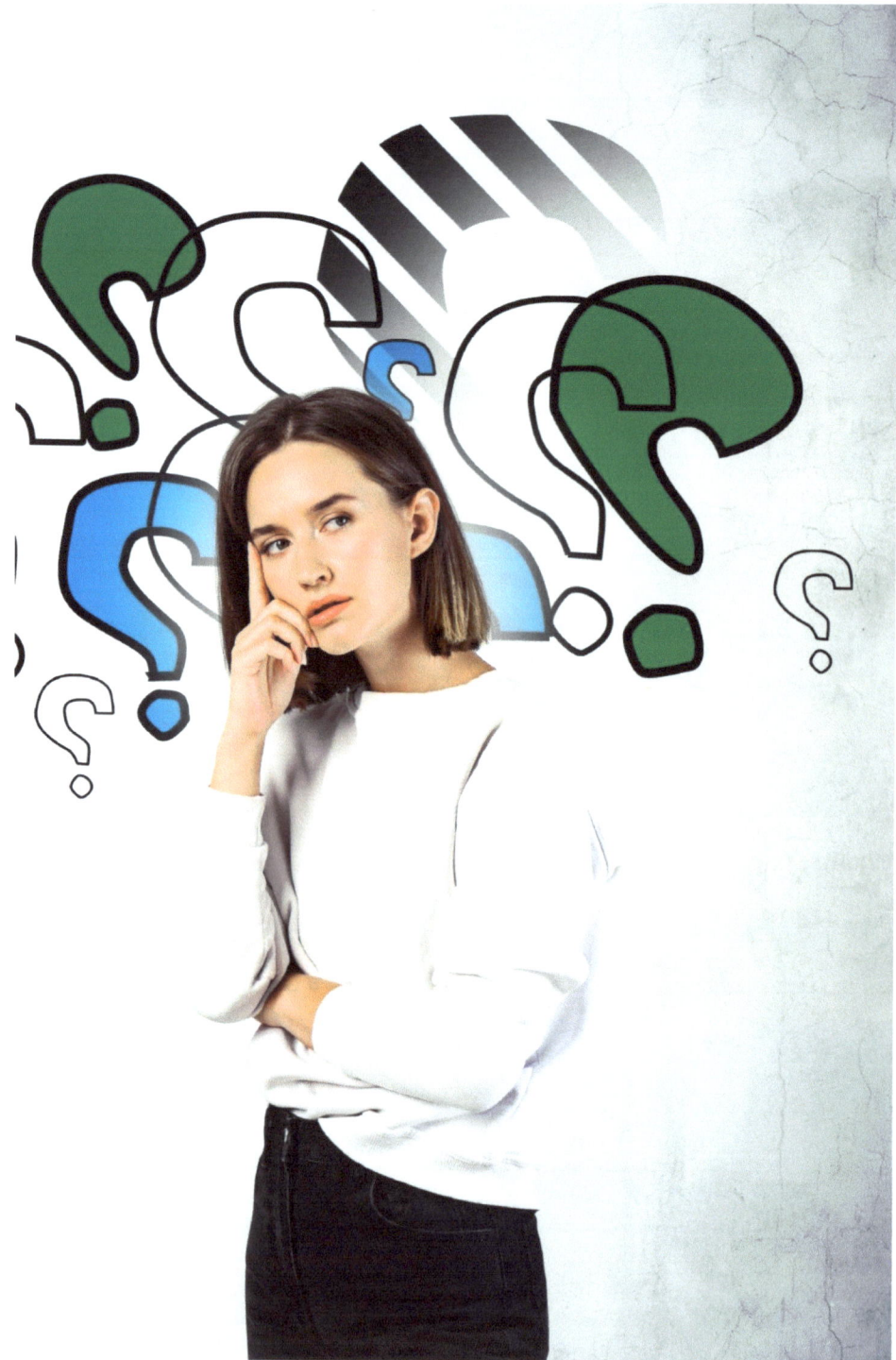

Day 6

How do you describe your path of spiritual development to this point?

- What do I value most in my life?
- What qualities do I most love and admire about myself? Why?
- How have they served me?

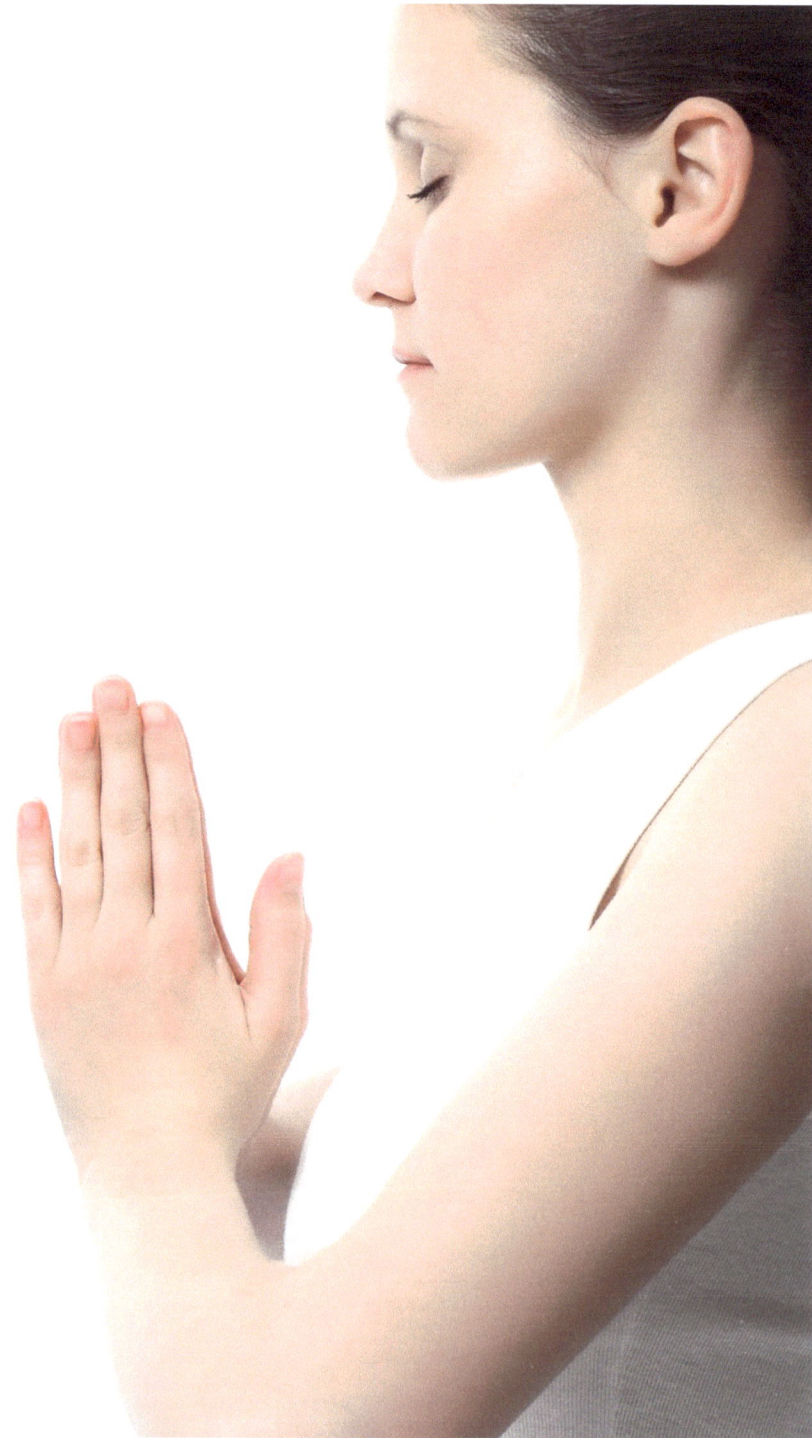

Day 7

Dreams are the doorway to the soul.

- What is a recent dream I had?
- What are the top 3 priorities in my life right now - why are they important to me?
- How do I honor them?
- If I had all the courage and support I would _____

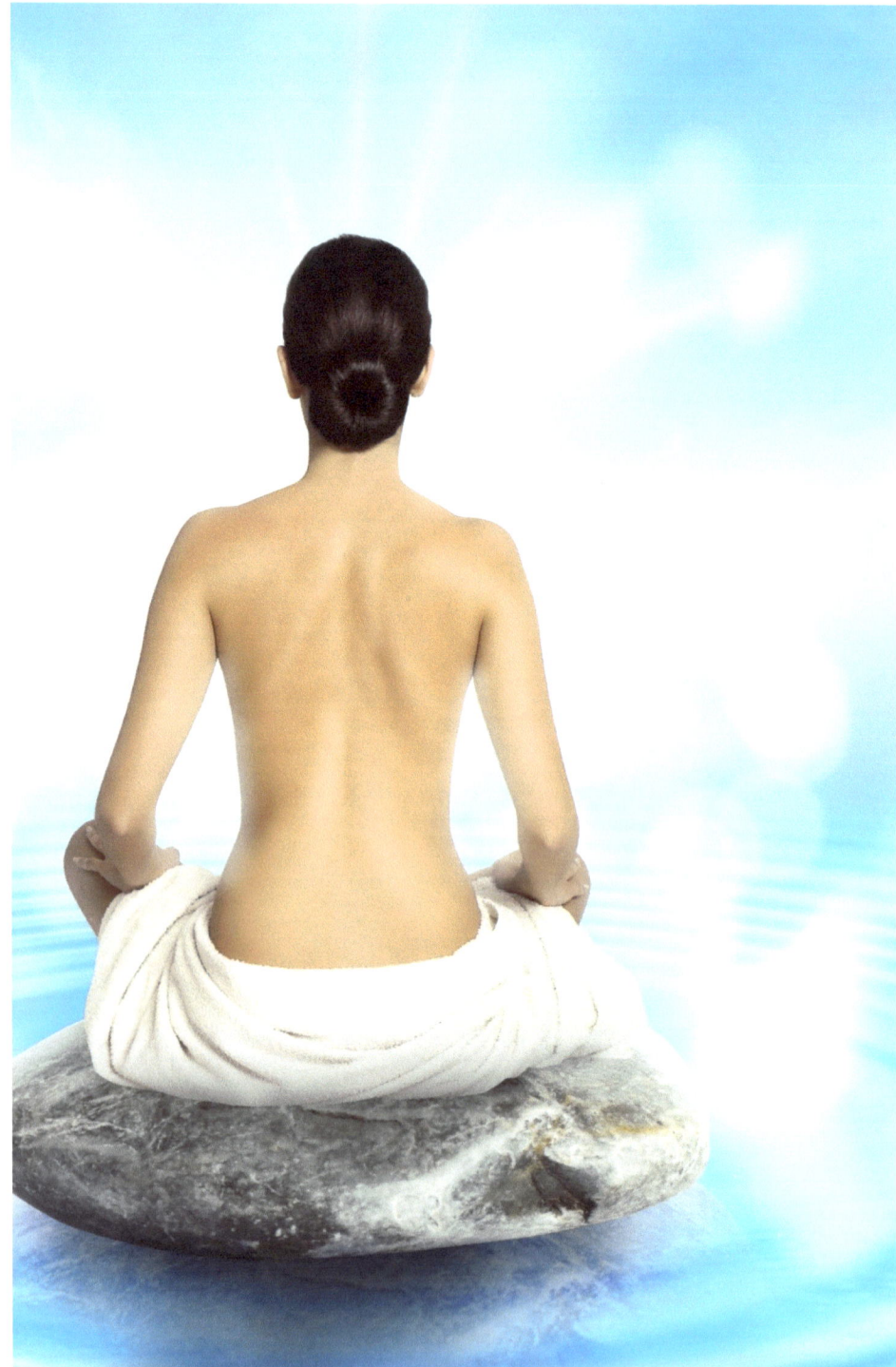

Day 8

Find a picture of yourself as a child.

- What did I dream about at that age?
- What were the highlights of my life - the low-lights?
- What are the lessons in each?
- Who or what drains my energy?
- What am I to do about it?

What do I choose to hold to and what do I want to let go?

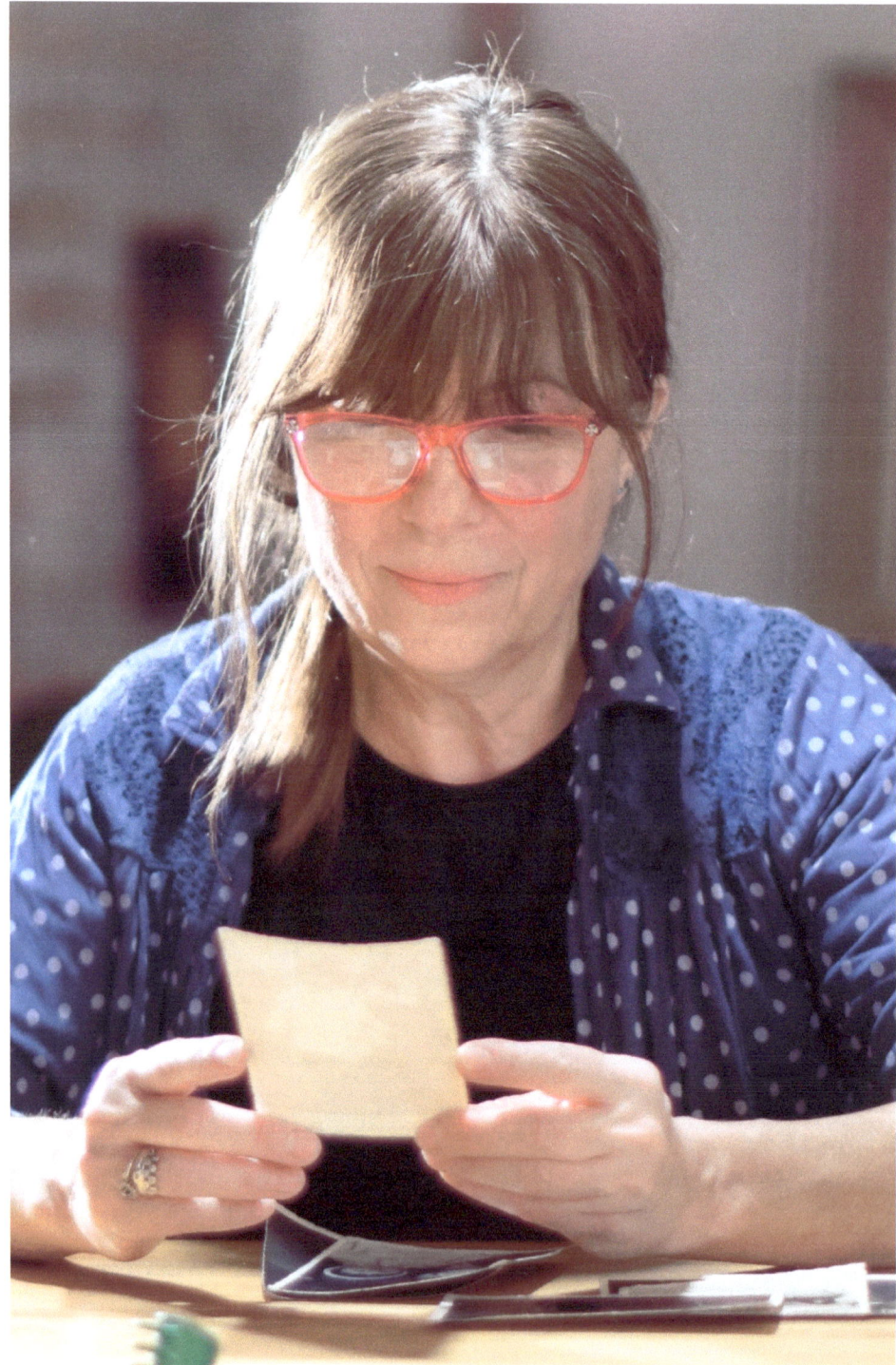

Day 9

Recall a favorite memory.

- What does this memory remind me of - what makes this memory special?
- If I had a chance to trade places for a day, which would it be?
- How do I feel about this memory now?

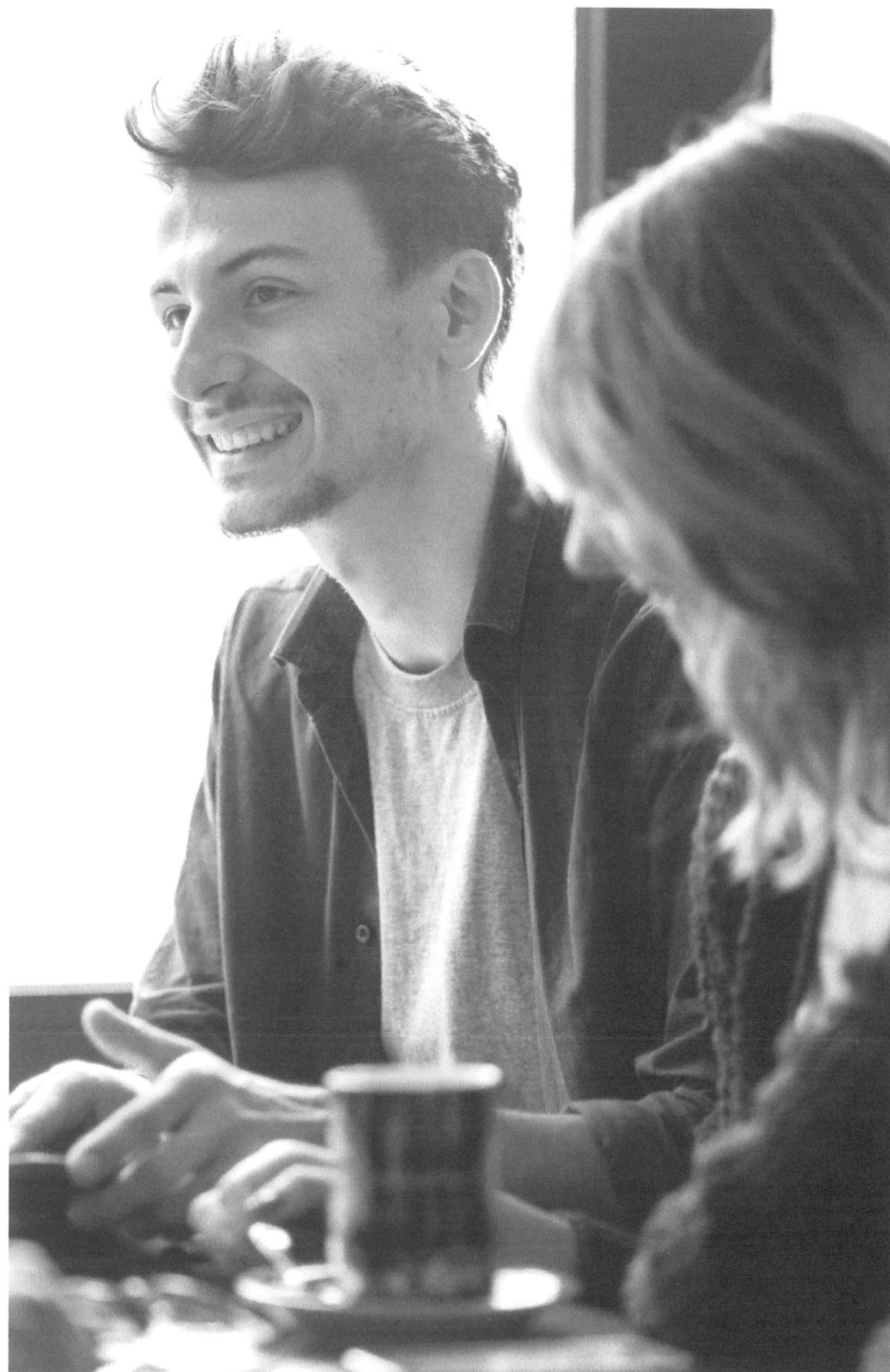

Day 10

Think of a time that you were most courageous and emotionally strong.

- What strengths did I have?
- Which can I call upon?
- How has this experience influenced me?
- If I could alter or relieve an incident in my life, which one would it be?
- What would I do differently today?

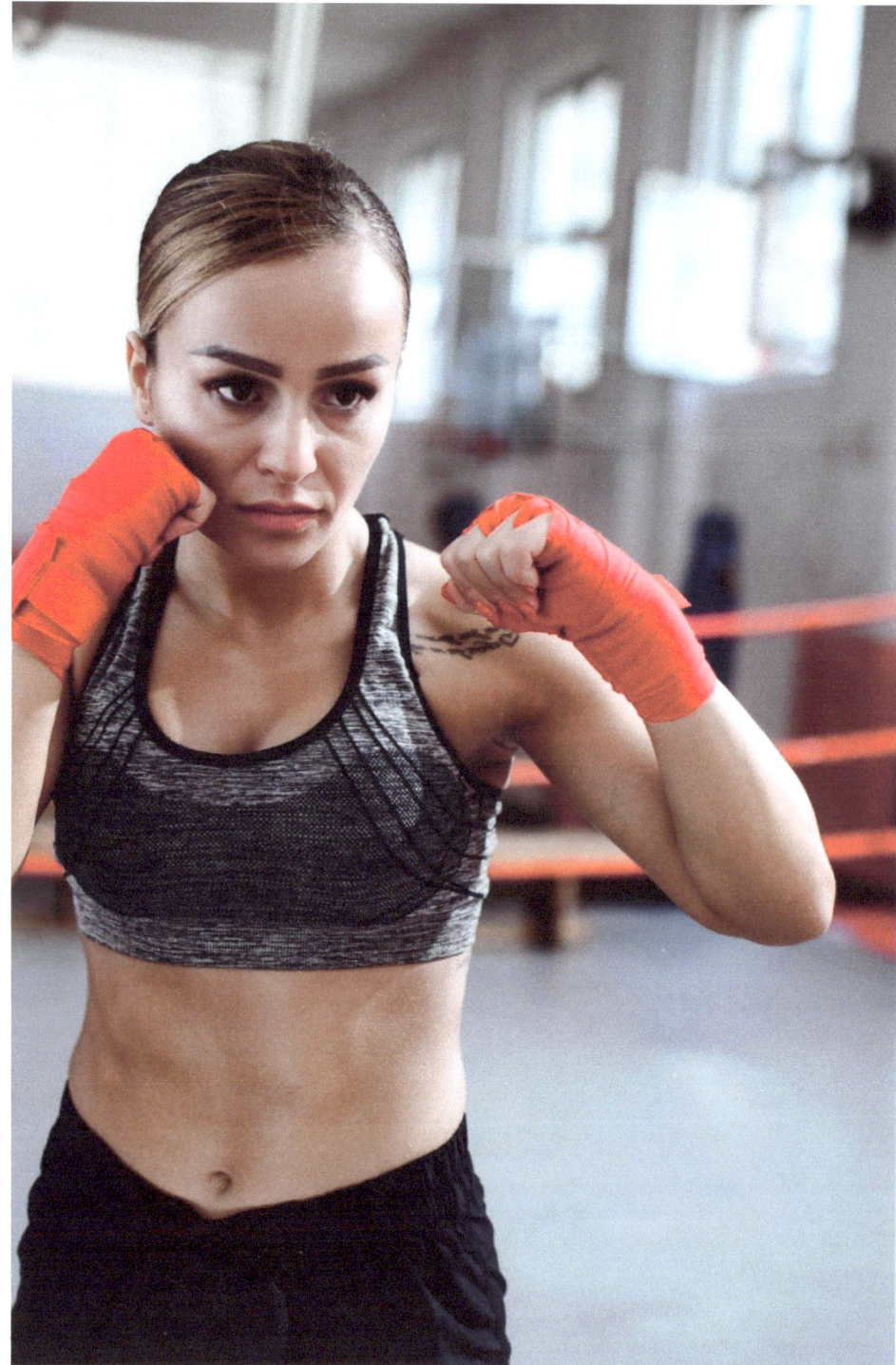

Day 11

What 3 words define how you engage and treat others?

- What blessings do I need today?
- How might they serve me?
- How would my life be any different?

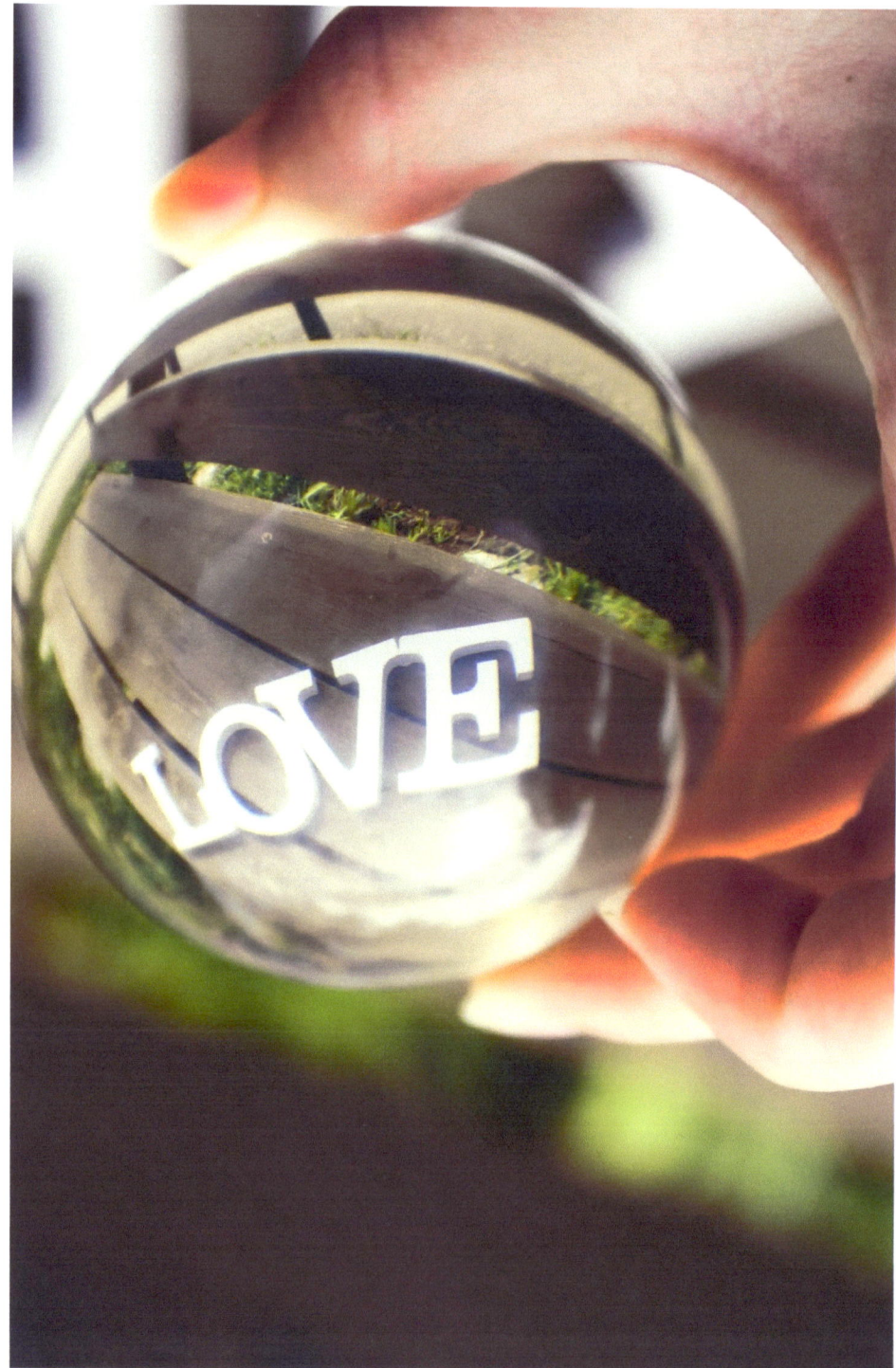

Day 12

How do you feel loved?

- When did I first experience falling in love? What was it like?
- How do I feel loved by someone?
- How do I define love?
- What does love mean to me now?
- How have my views on love changed over the years?

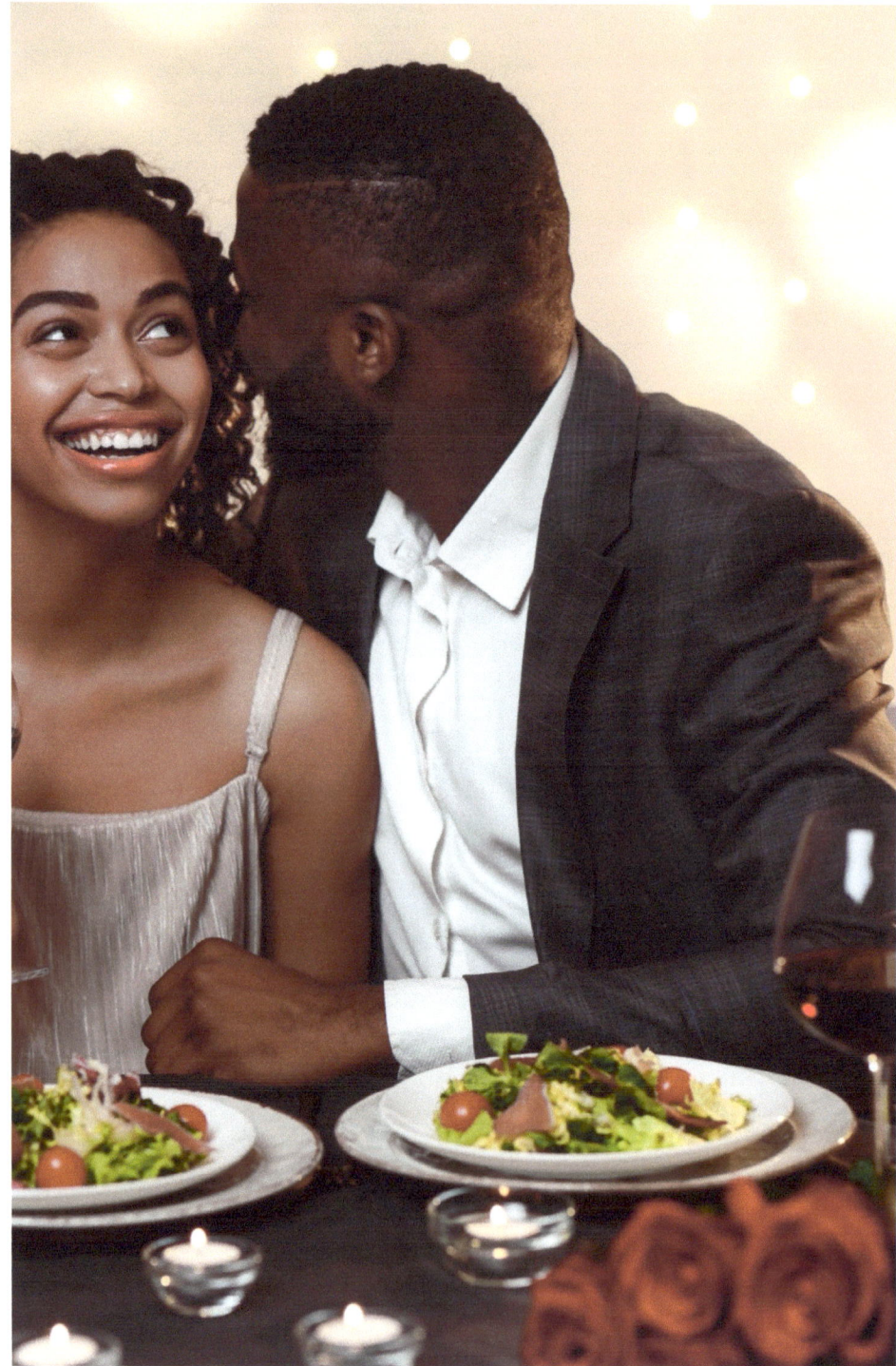

Day 13

When you look back over your life, family, or romantic relationships...

- What patterns or themes can I identify?
- Who were the important people in my life then and now?
- What do I admire or love the most about them?

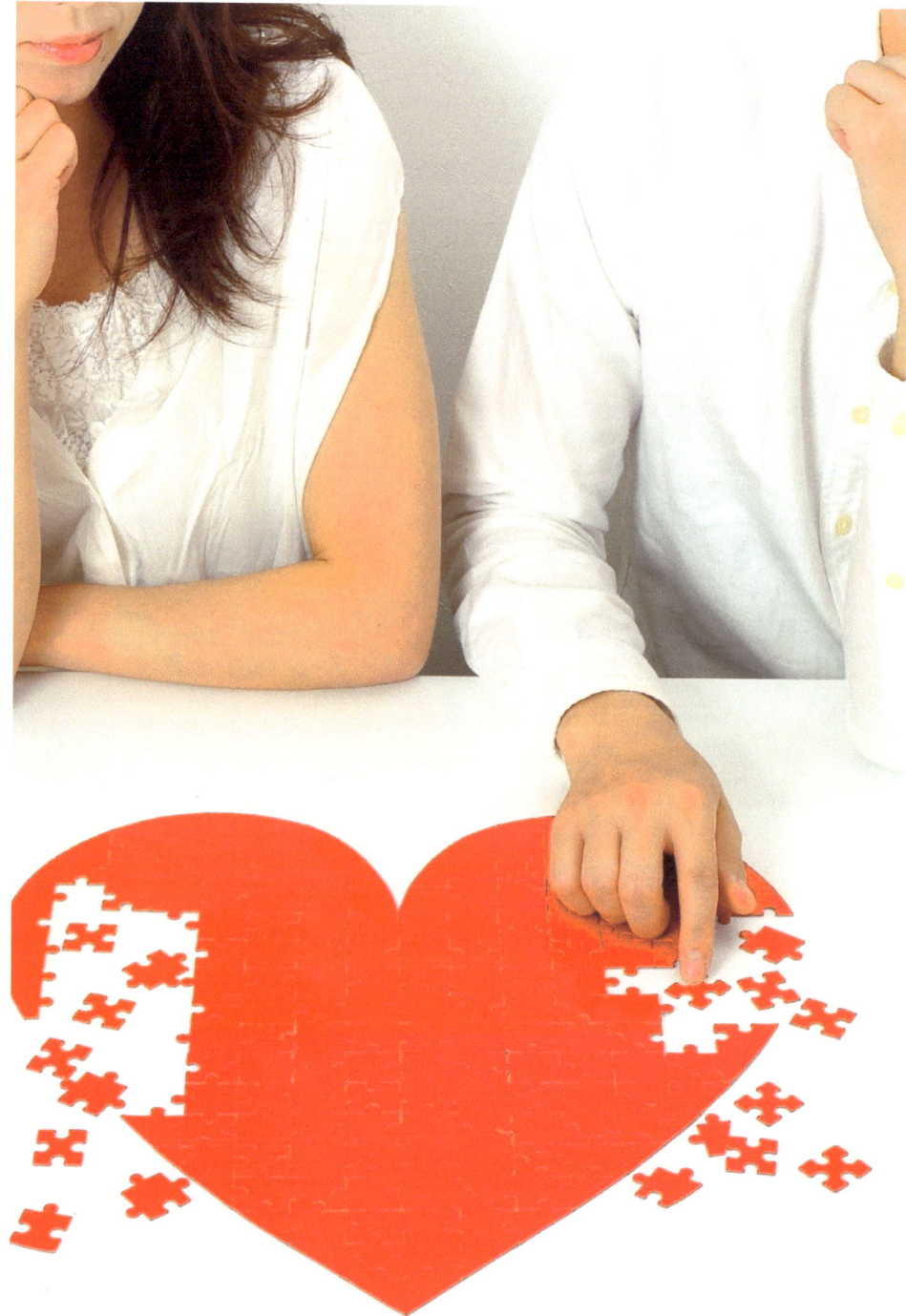

Day 14

How have you grown over the last year?

- What qualities have I developed to strengthen my character?
- What is my personal style?
- What is the mood or tone I want to project?
- What are my best qualities?
- What qualities do I need to develop?
- How do I cultivate them?

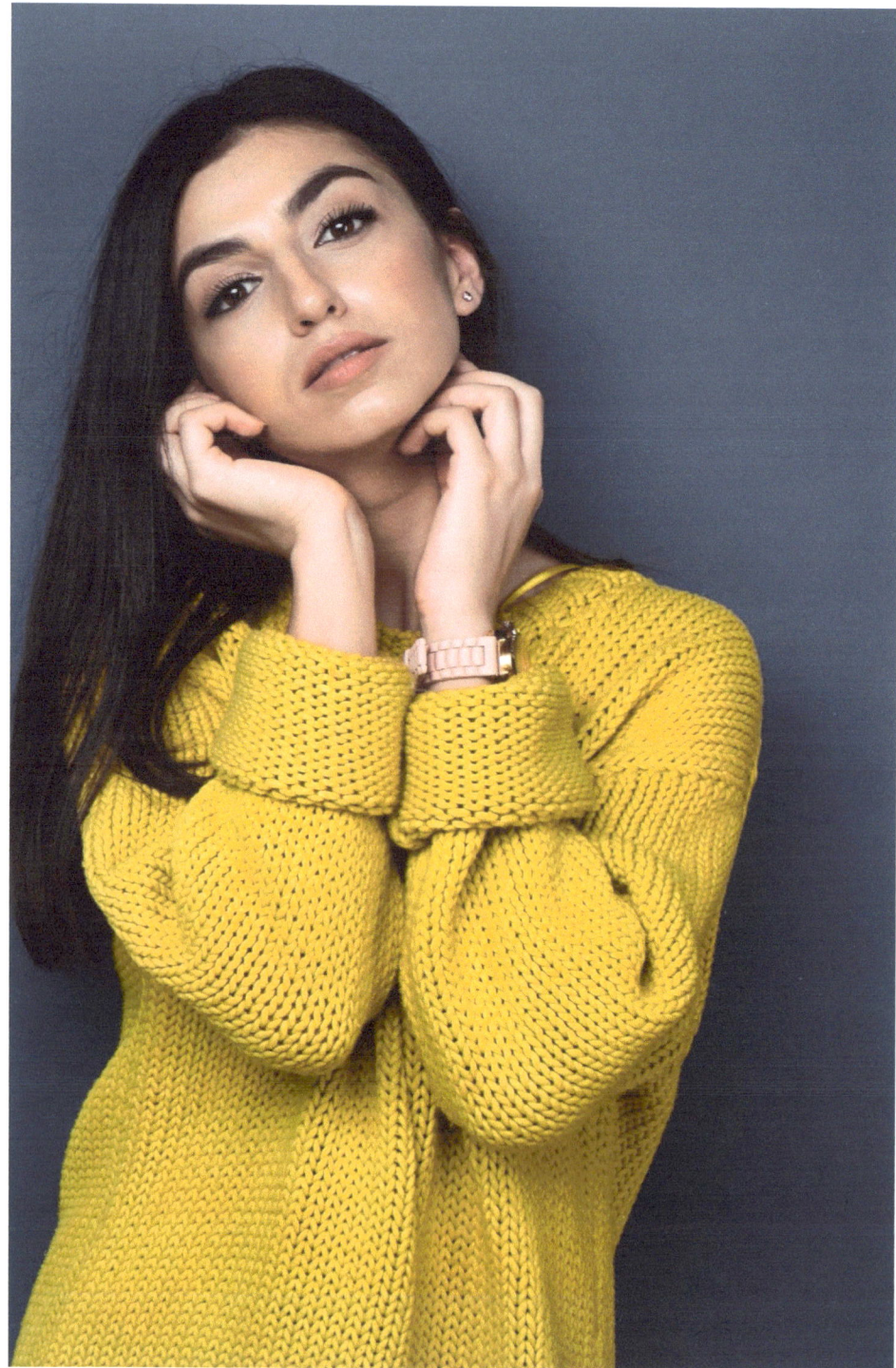

Day 15

List some of your favorite books, magazines.

- What do I like to read?
- What do they have in common?
- Why is this genres interest me?
- How are they enhancing my way of thinking, being, living?
- What have I learned from them?

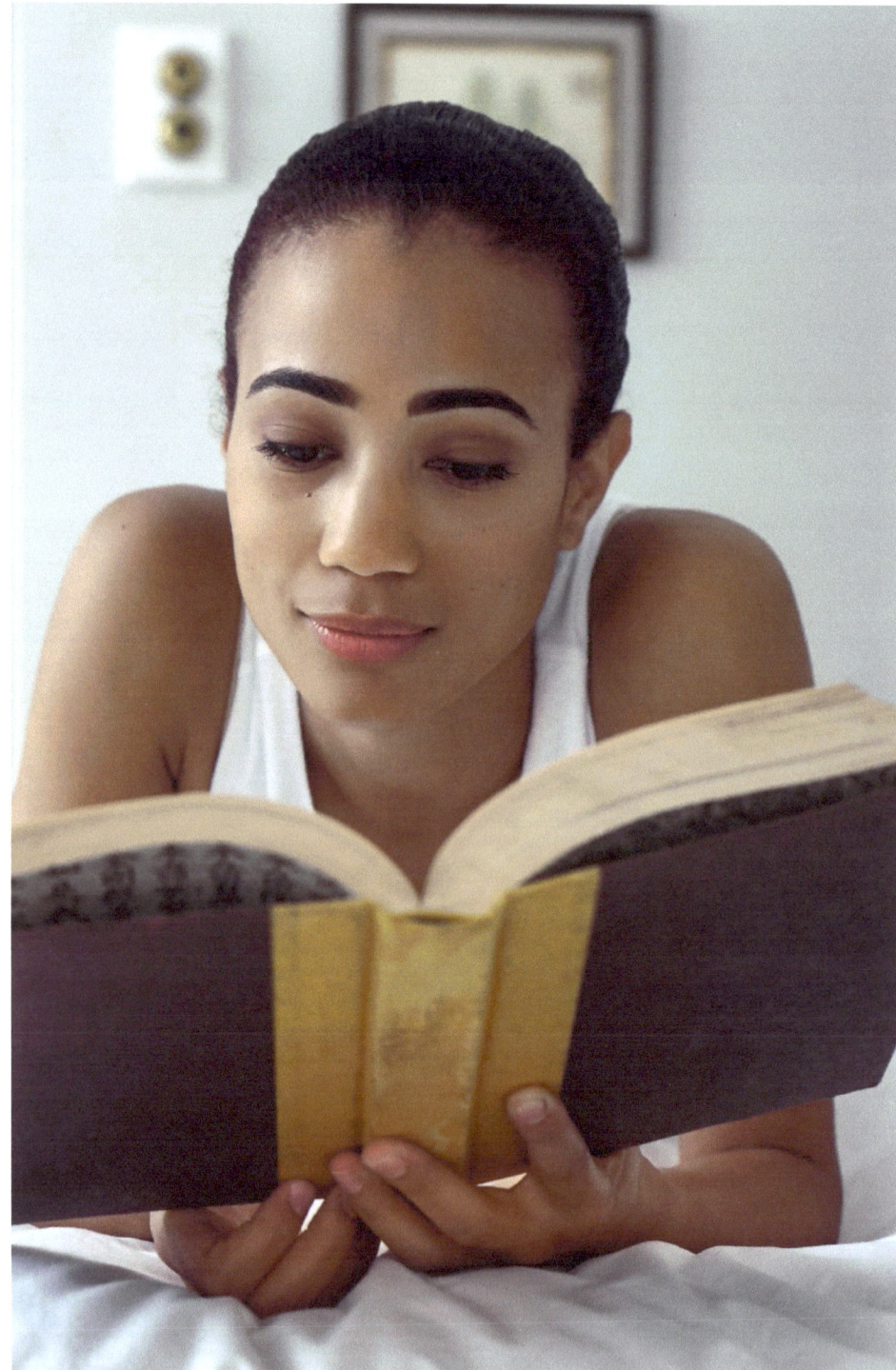

Day 16

How do you improve your health?

- What do I crave the most?
- What foods do I gravitate to in which I comfort myself when I am upset, sad, lonely, tired, or overwhelmed?
- Do I use food to make me feel good?
- If I become more mindful, how would my lifestyle be any different?

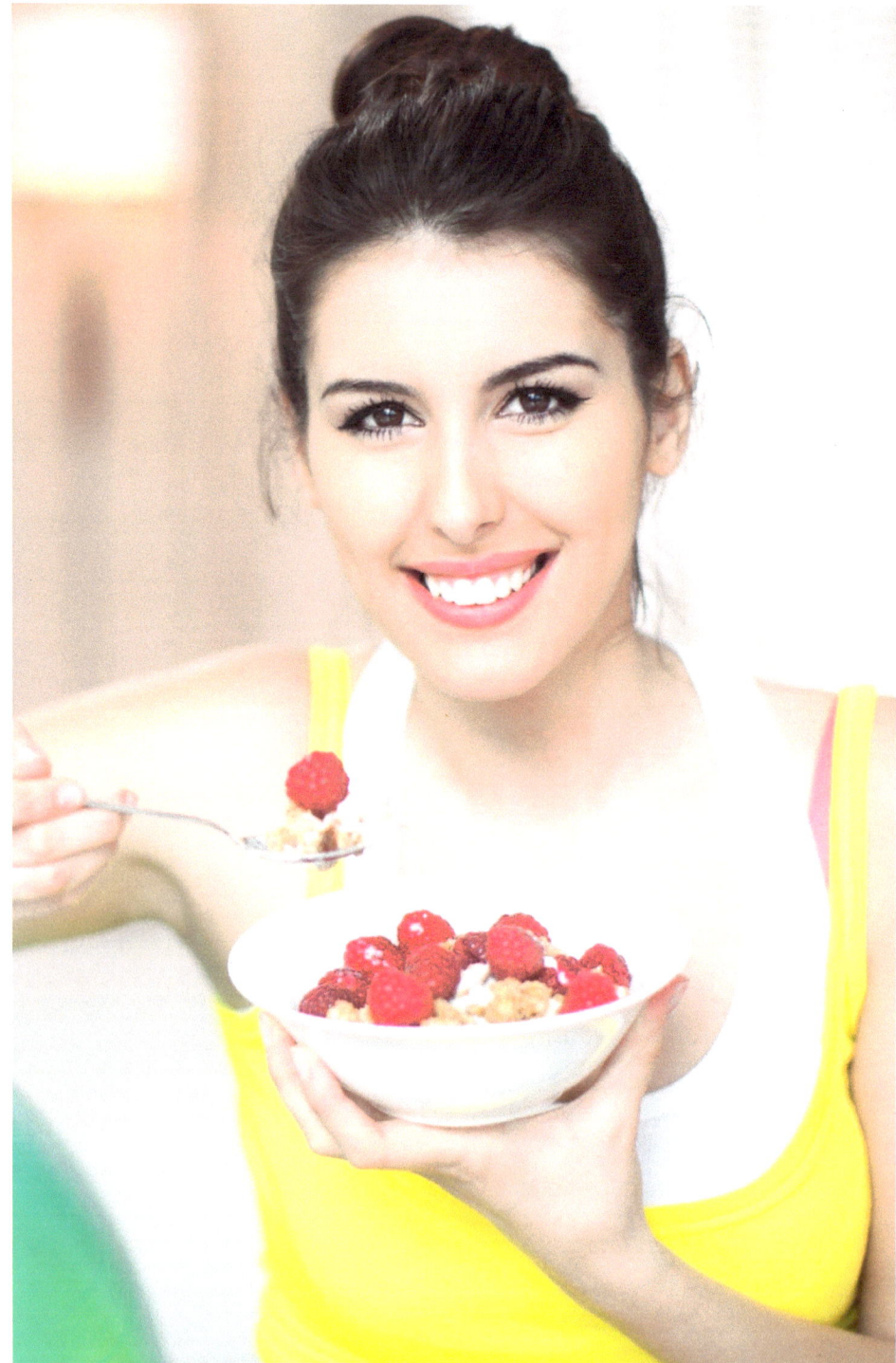

Day 17

Create an abundance list to see the blessings you receive each day.

- What message did I learn growing up about money and wealth?
- What is the message and attitude of my loved ones about money?
- How have these messages affected me in my adulthood?
- If I had all the money, time, confidence, and self-awareness in the world, how would my life be any different?
- Am I in a good place today?

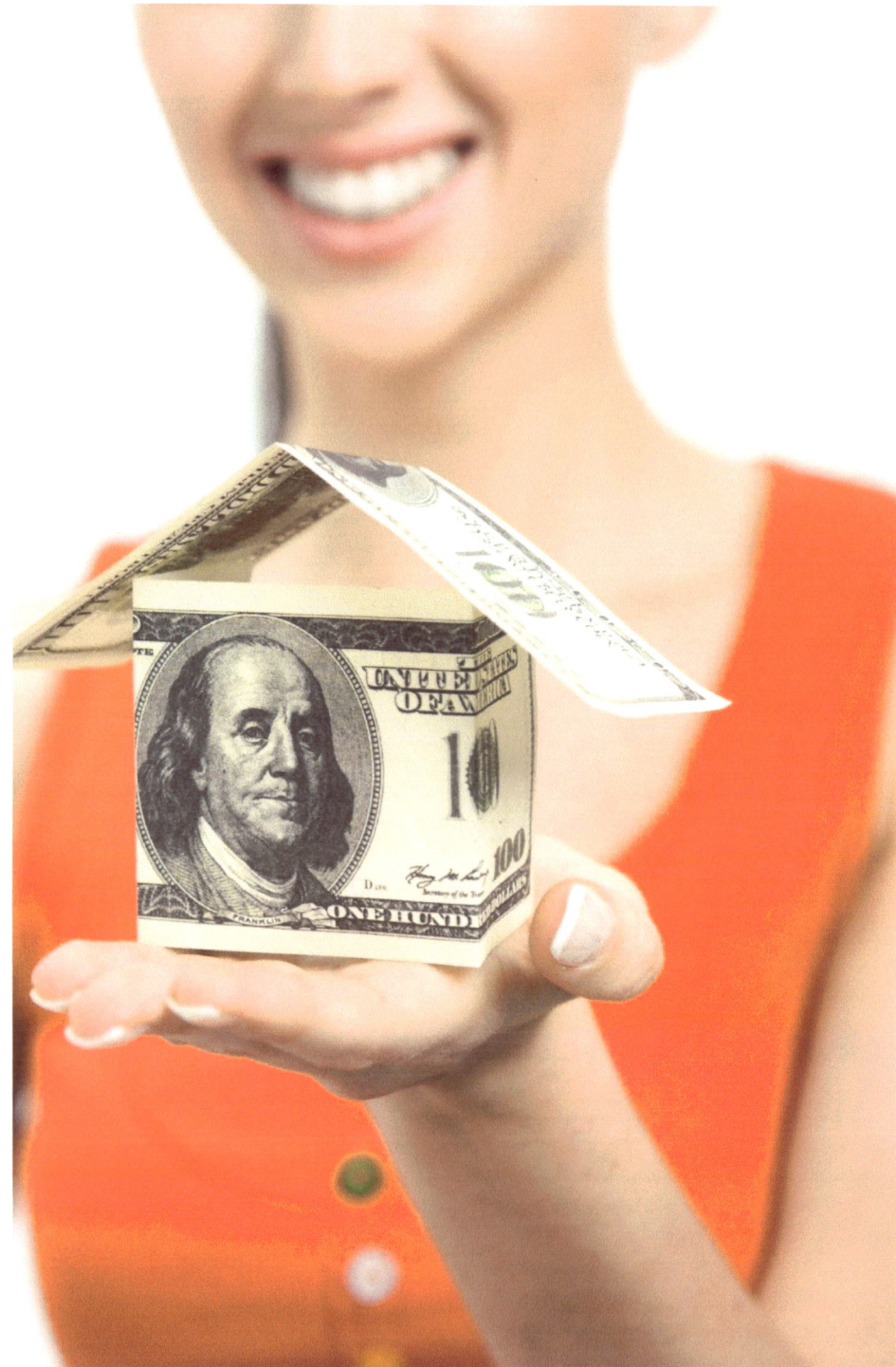

Day 18

What is your perfect vacation?

- Where did I dream of as a child?
- Where would I go now?
- How would I go?
- With whom?
- What would I do - or want to experience?

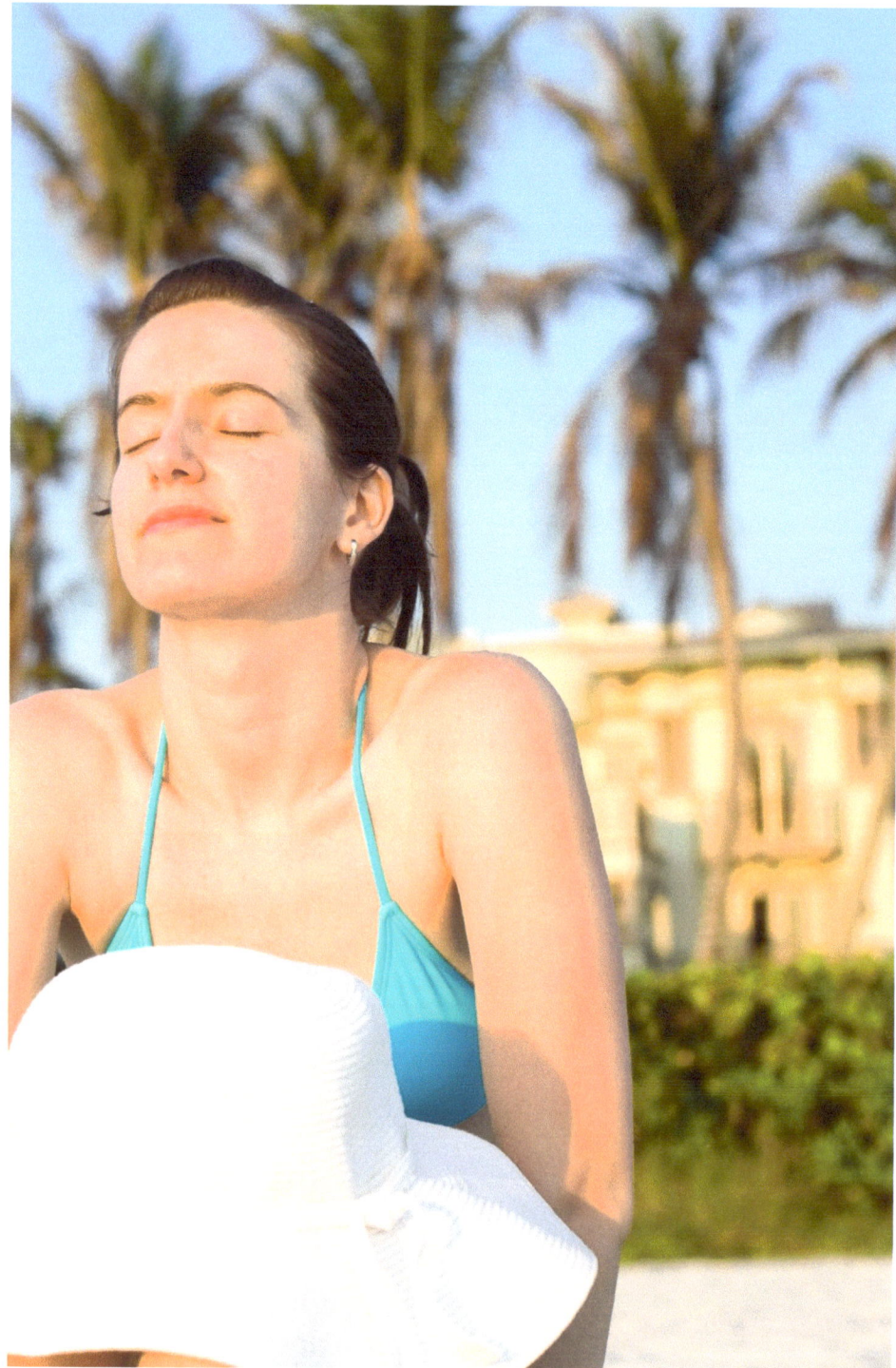

Day 19

What 3 boundaries do you need to set for yourself to create the space for more success in life - personally and professionally?

- What do I need for myself to feel more secure?
- How would I respond if someone were to ask me:
  - Who are you
  - What do you want?
  - What do you need?

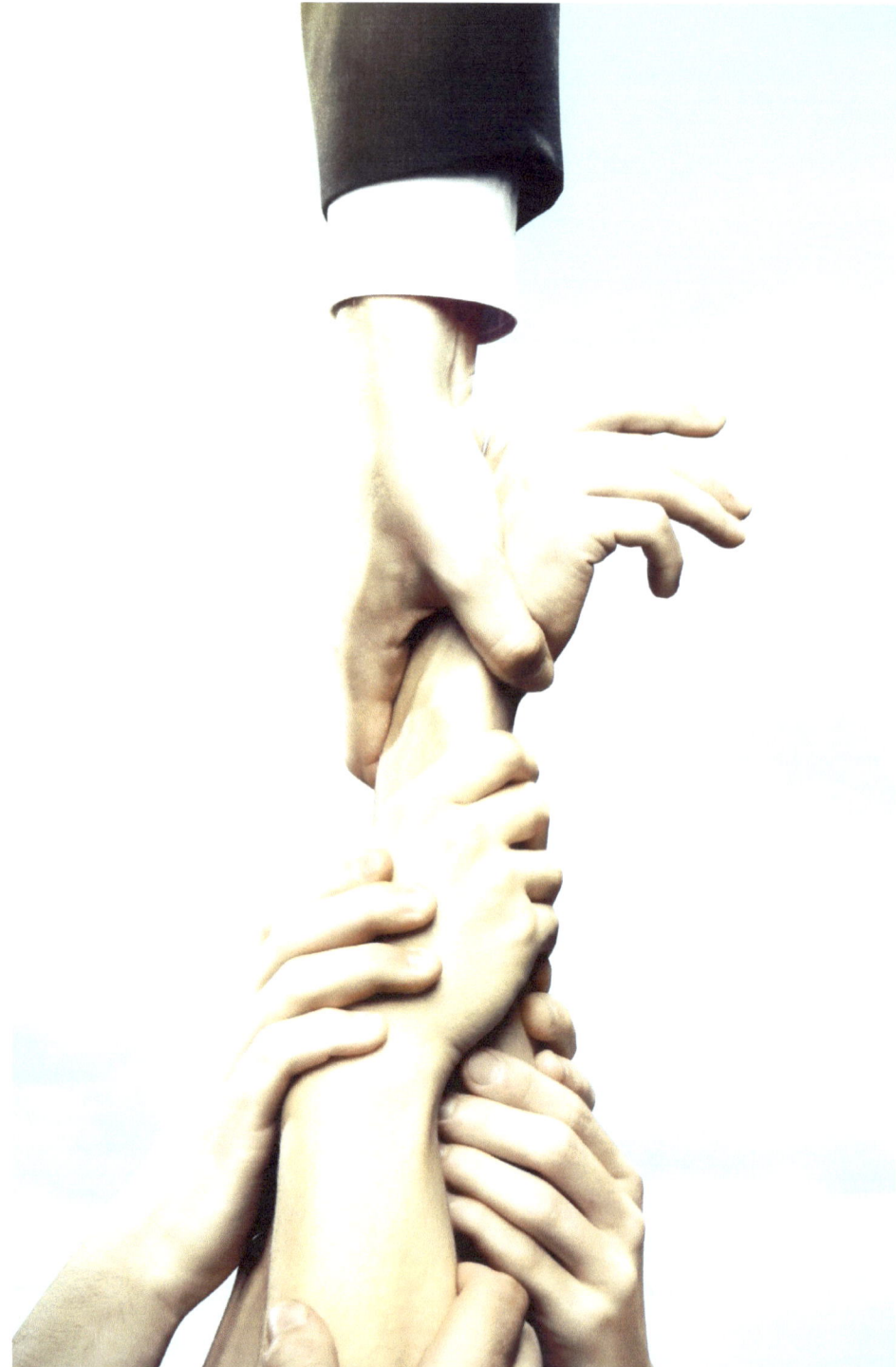

Day 20

As you decide to use your talents
and gifts in an even greater way,
what would you do differently?

- How do I show up in life?
- What do I want to project to
others?
- How am I seen?
- What 15 skills do I possess?

Review the list and circle the ones
you love most.

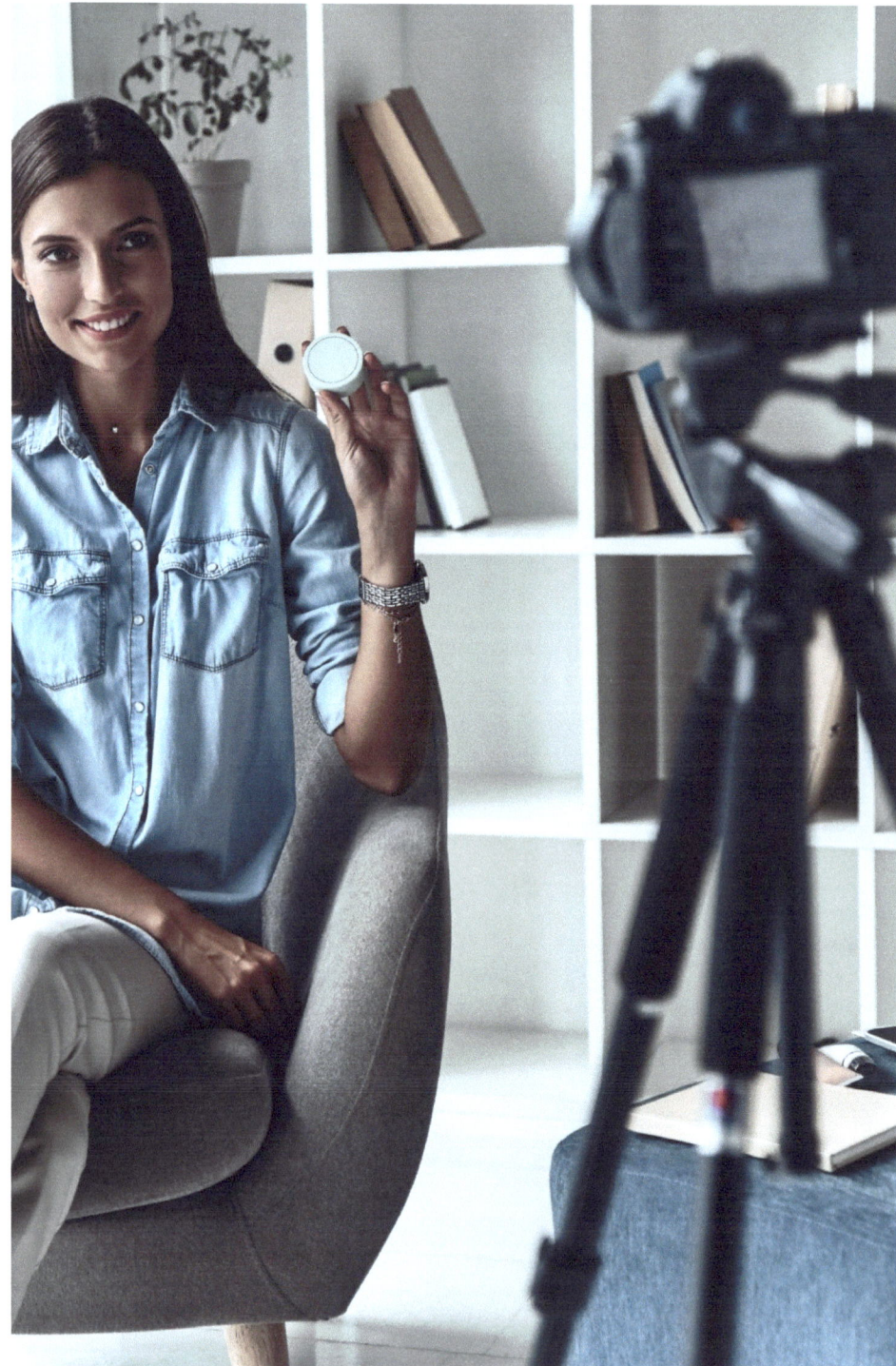

Day 21

How can you hone your skills better and make use of them?

- What do I want?
- What do I need?
- What might my inner self be wanting to remind or tell me?

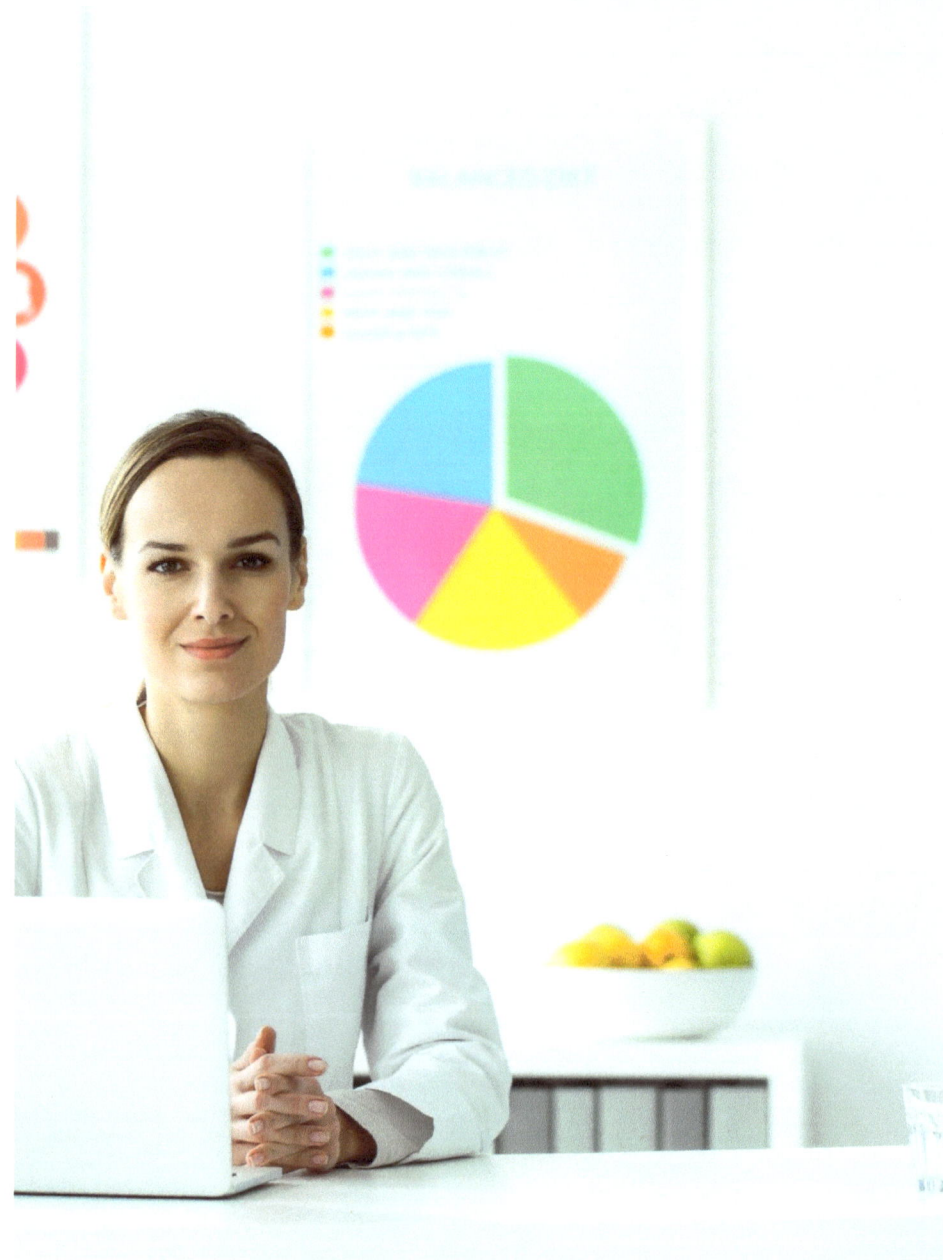

Day 22

Interview 3 close friends or family members - ask them to describe the qualities that make you unique and special.

• Am I willing and open to hear their honest opinion?
• What would they say?
• What are my special gift?
• What are my not so good habits and traits?
• What did I learn different about myself?

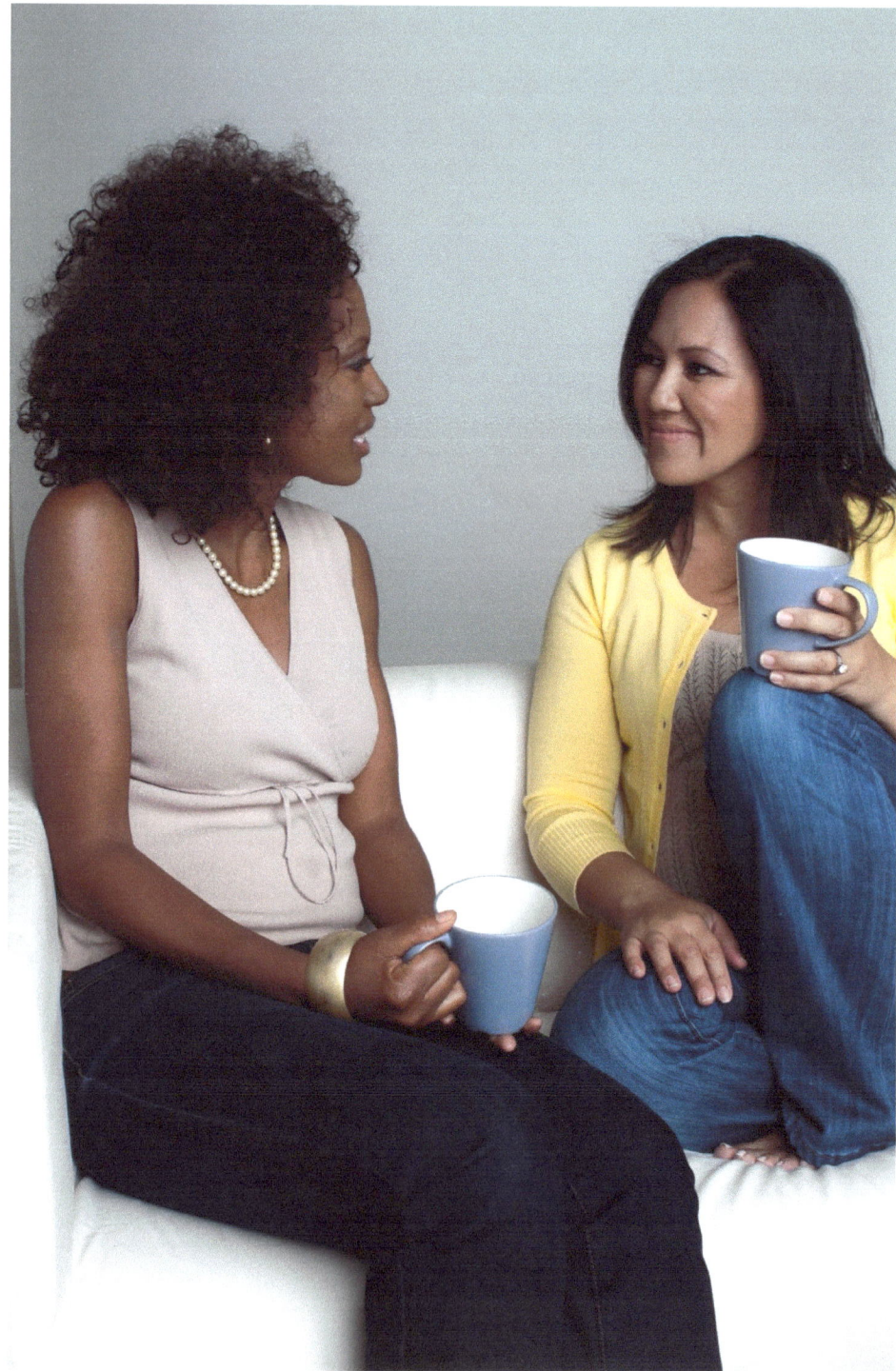

Day 23

What do you dream about doing with your life?

- Is there anything stopping me?
- What do I aspire to accomplish?
- What legacy do I wish to leave for others?
- What bigger impact do I want to make in life?

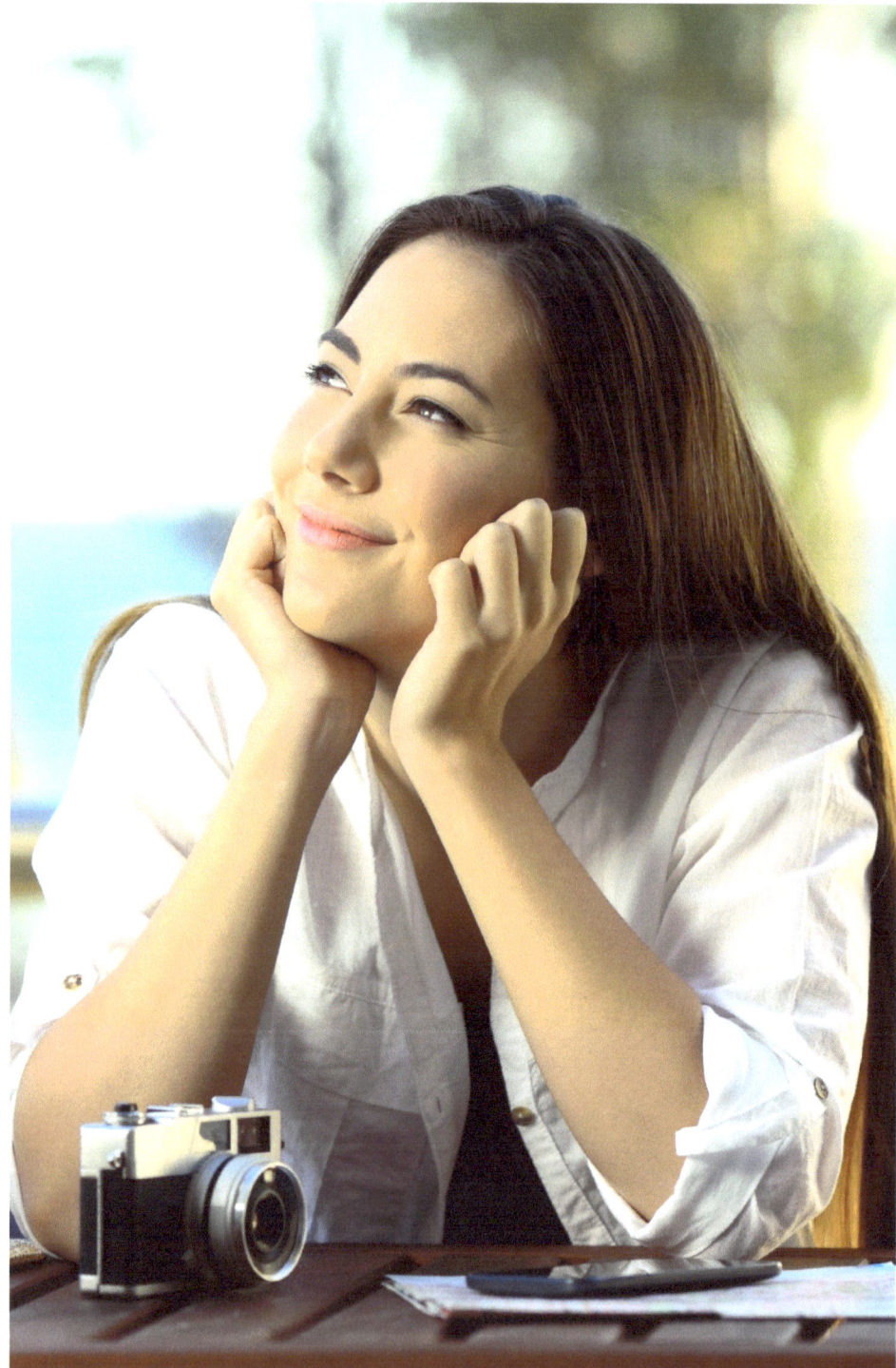

Day 24

Everything you do today is a reflection of what you are ready to embrace.

What 3 things do you need to guide you to the next level?
My burning desire is _____
I am ready to cultivate a new mindset
I desire freedom in mind and body
I desire self expression
I embrace all that I am
I desire to Show Up and Speak Up!

Nothing in life happens without grace

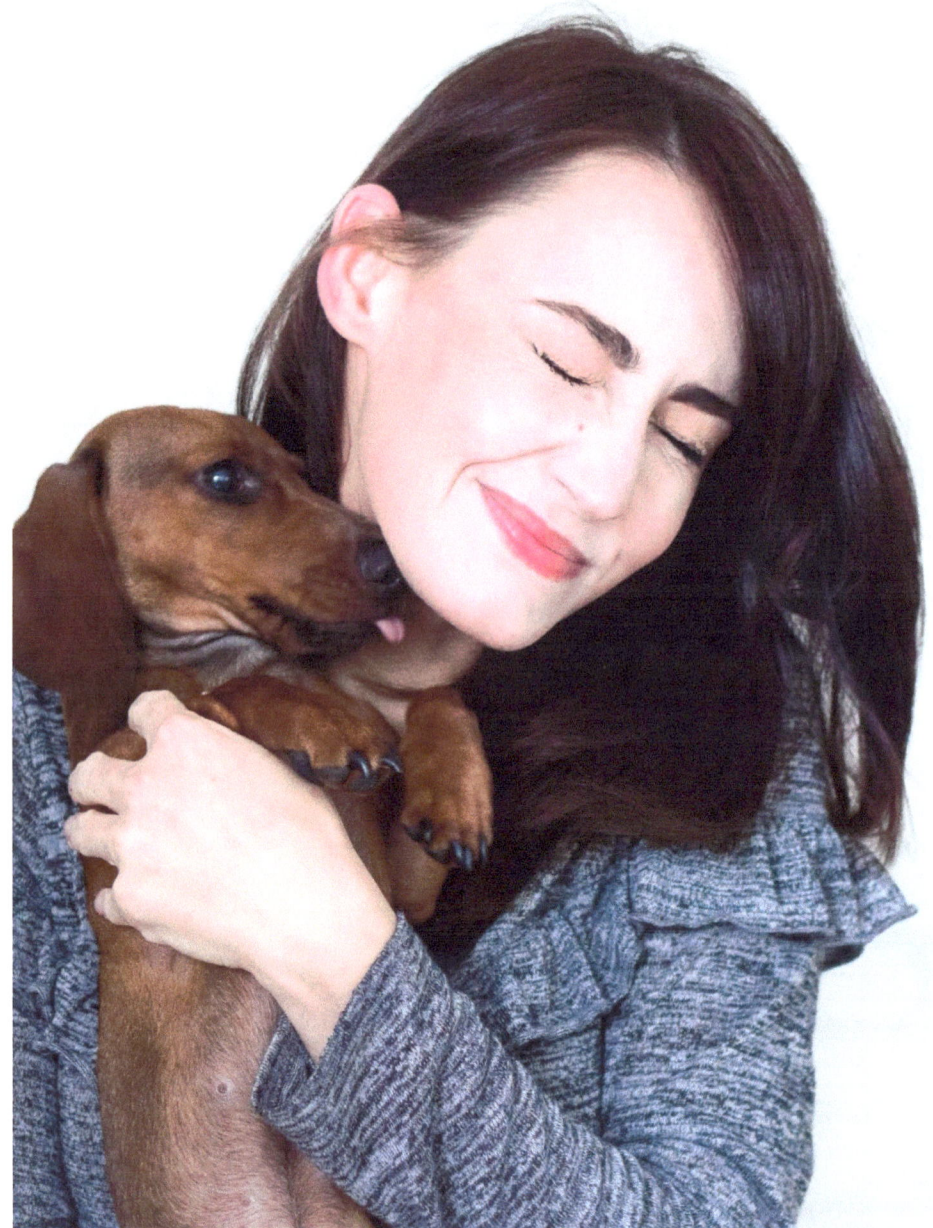

Day 25

When your expectation is met,
that becomes a true essence of
who you are.

- Instead of making the best
  decision, I decide, and take
  ownership of that decision.
- I realize this decision is the best
  decision for now.
- I allow myself to receive.
- I attract abundance into my life.

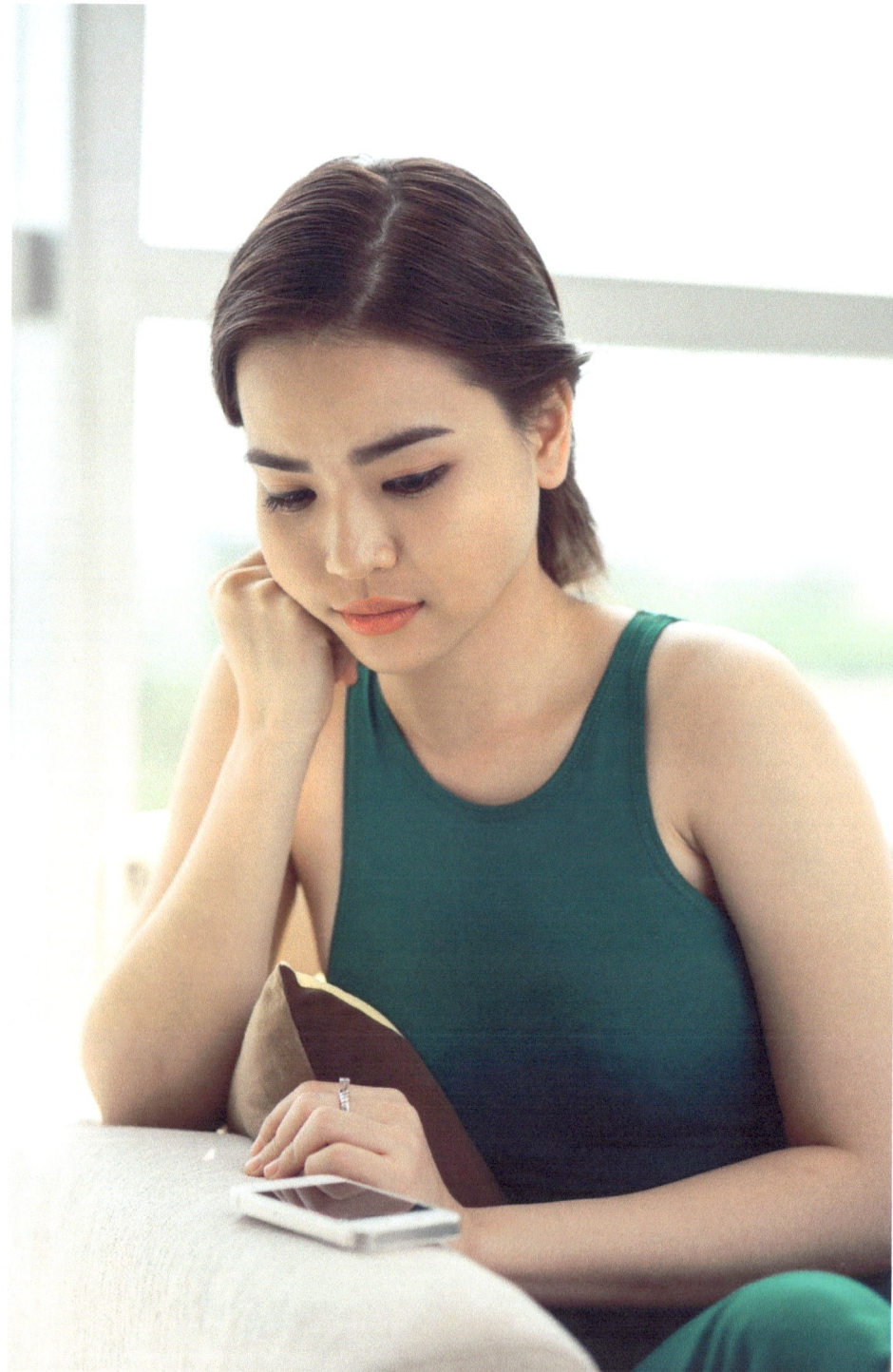

Day 26

Pausing for a moment in life.

I slow down, I pause, and I choose to enjoy the environment I am in.

When I pause for a moment, I breathe for my body.

I am thankful for everything that surrounds me.

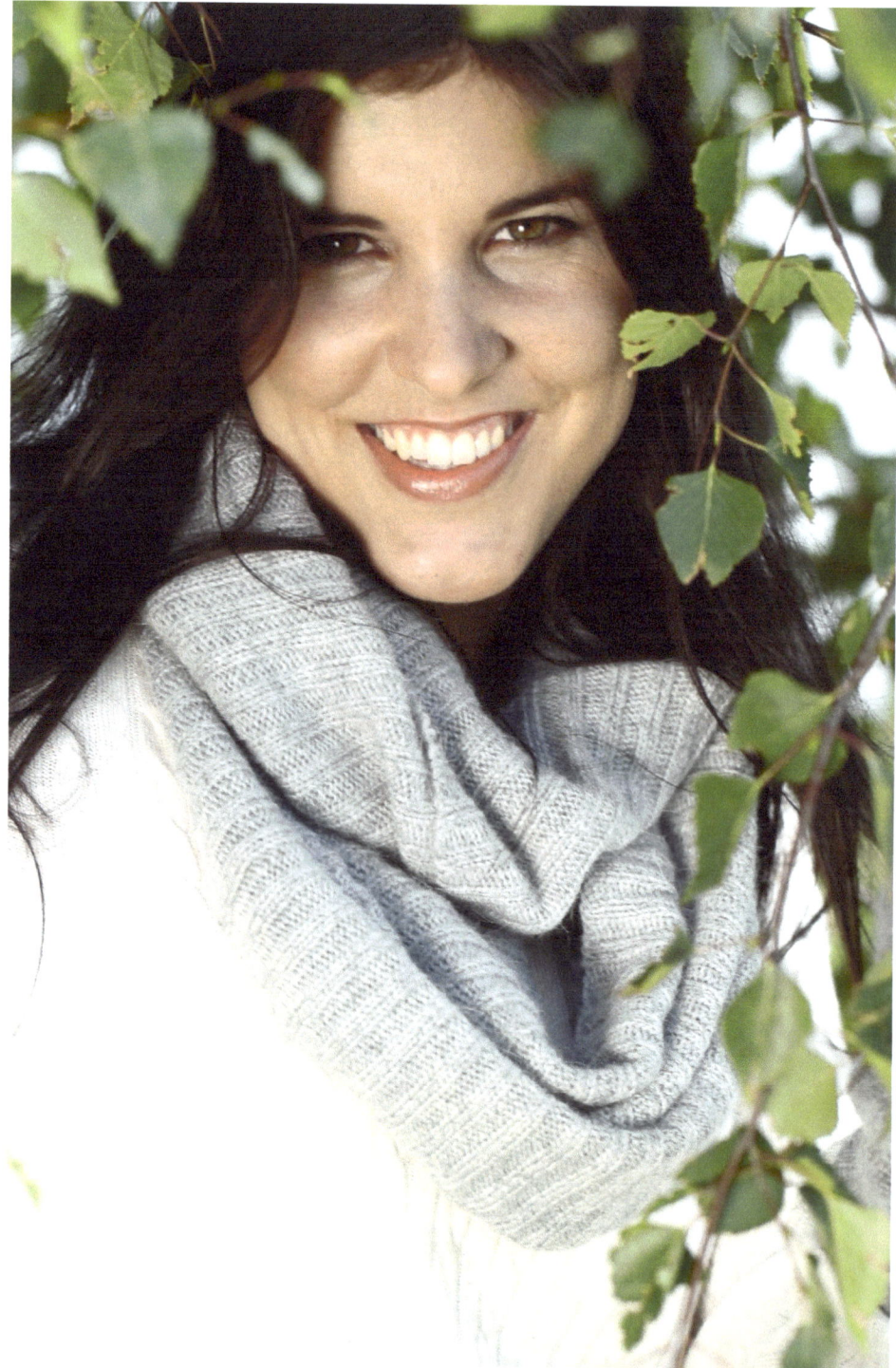

Day 27

Observe - write down 100 things you like or love that you have surrounded yourself with.

Start your sentences with:
I Feel - I Will - I Can - I Choose - I Want

I choose positive words that empower and move me to feelingl better and more confident.

Confidence is defined as "I AM"

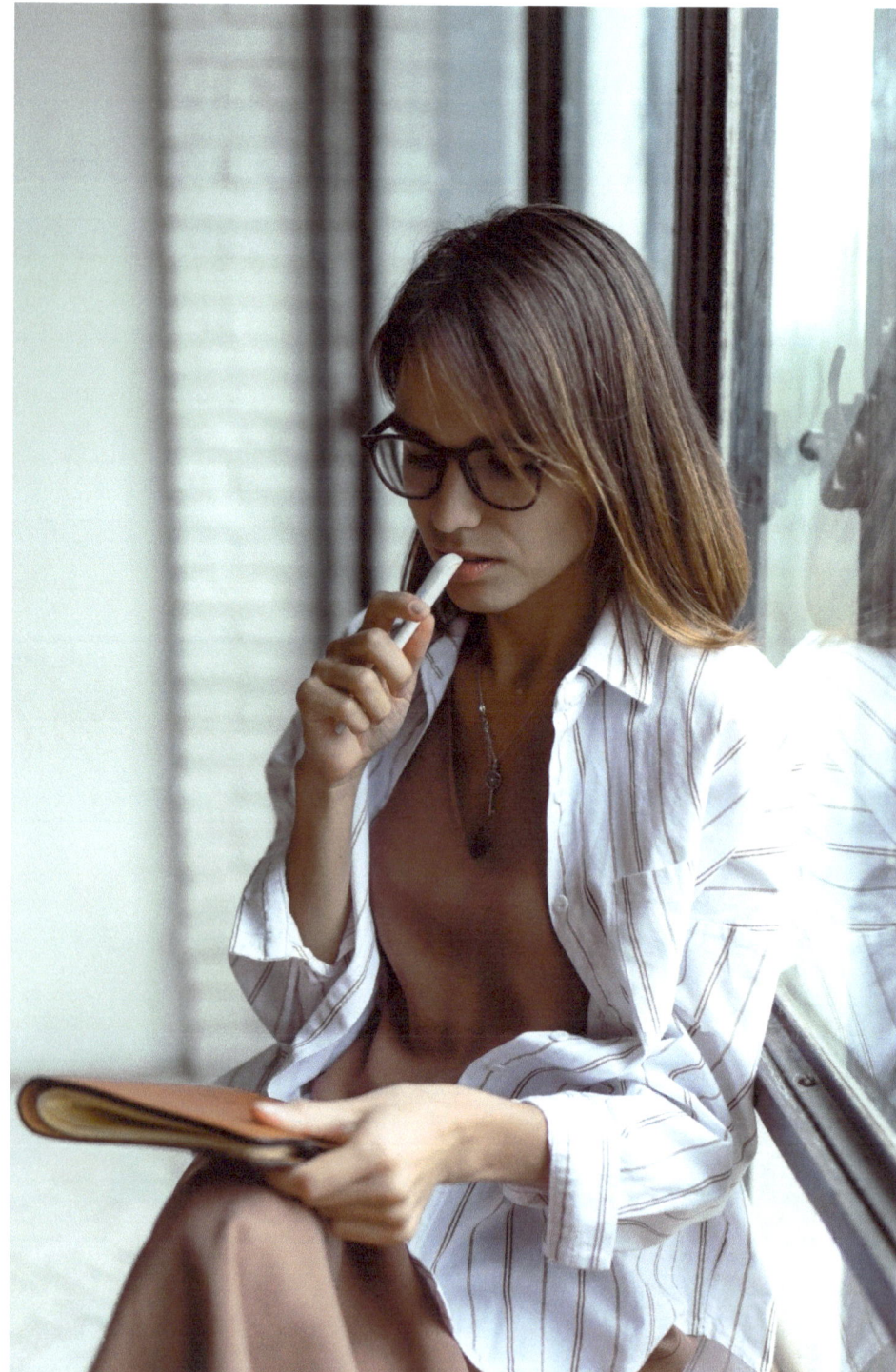

Day 28

Every experience has been a part of your learning process.

What experiences in my life can I:
– Forgive -
– See the lesson -
– Let go of -
– Keep and repeat -
– Be grateful to.

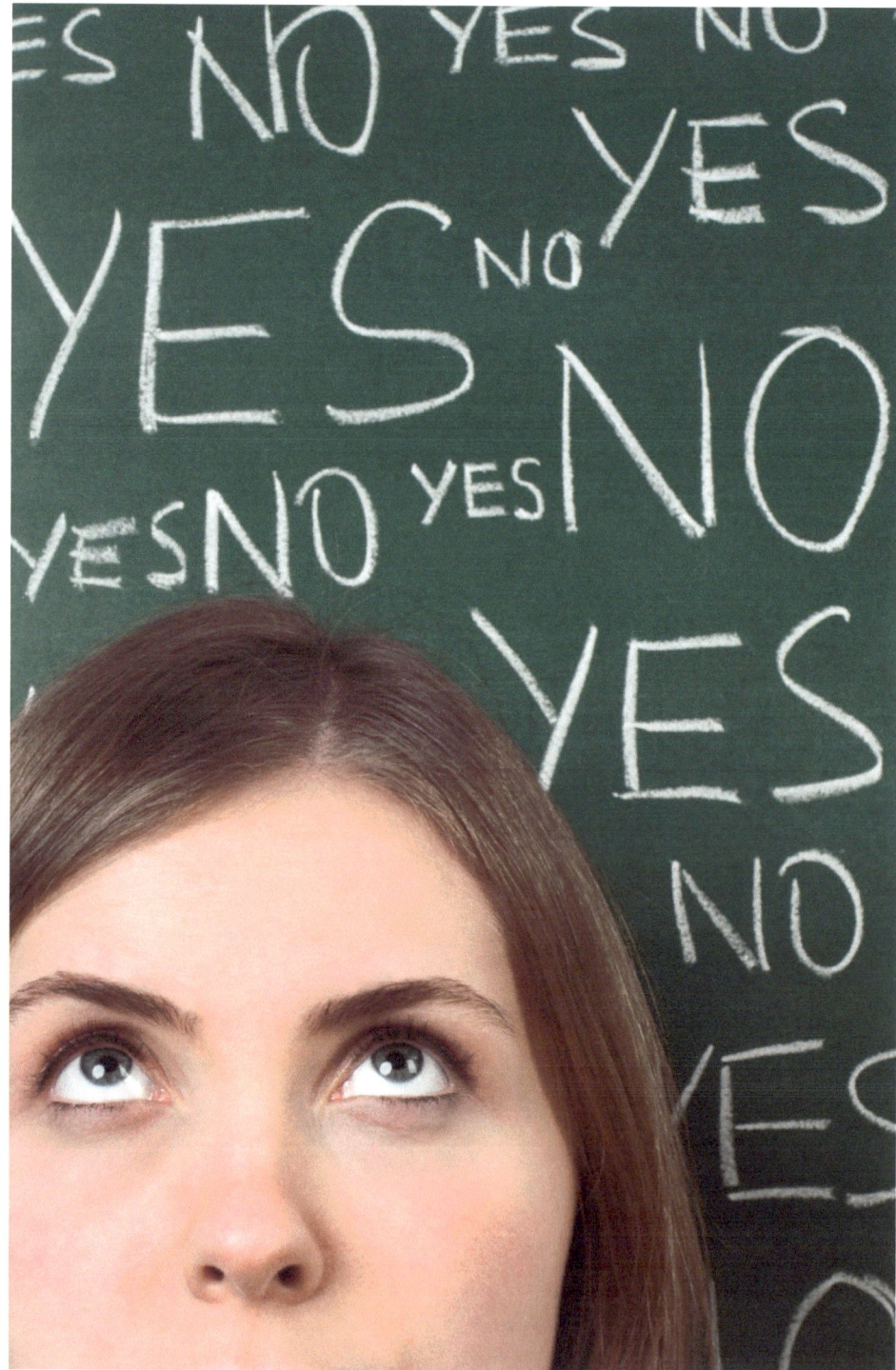

Day 29

What is one thing I can do today to embed and make these changes become consistent in me?

How would that change look like, sound like, feel like?

- YES - I'm ready to feel it, I'm ready to see it, I'm ready to BE it!
- I Matter!

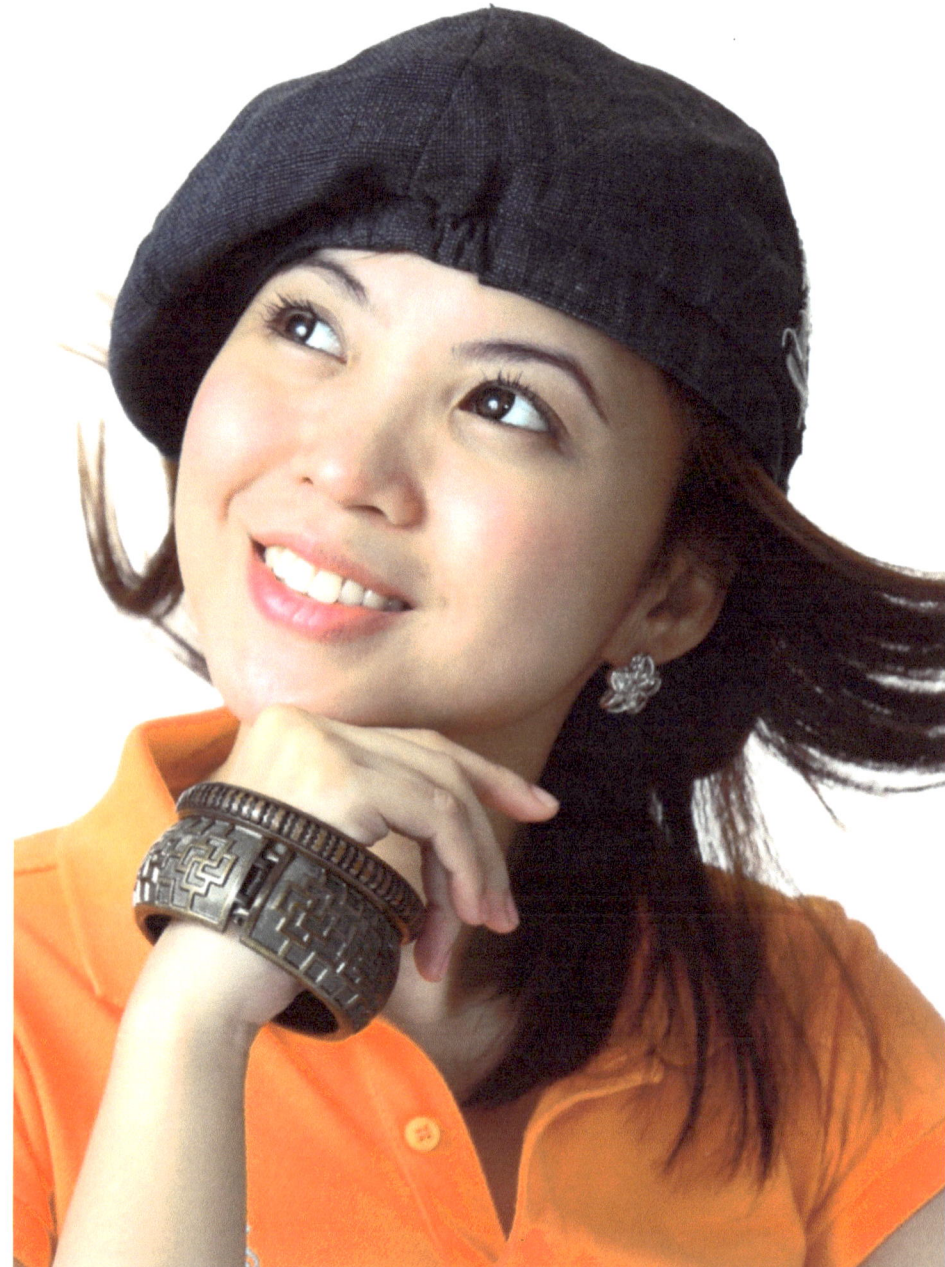

Day 30

Write a letter to God, a Higher Power, or the Universe.

- How have my thoughts changed because of completing this journal?
- Here is my own conversation with _____

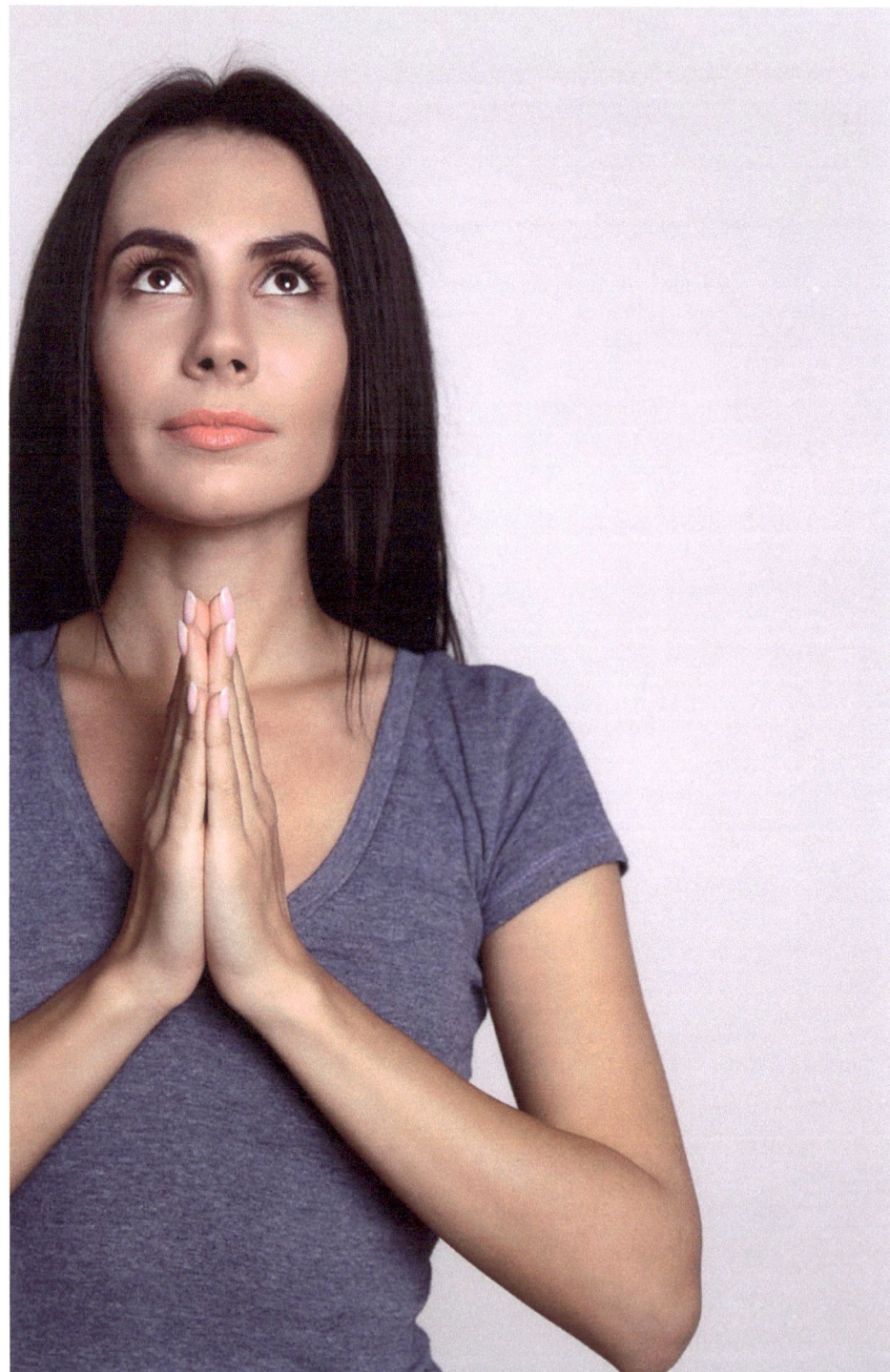

Day 31

I am excited and ready to immerse myself and evoke my desired goals.

- I See it,
- I Feel it,
- I Become It!
- It is ME~

Every day in every way, I accept and appreciate myself for who I AM

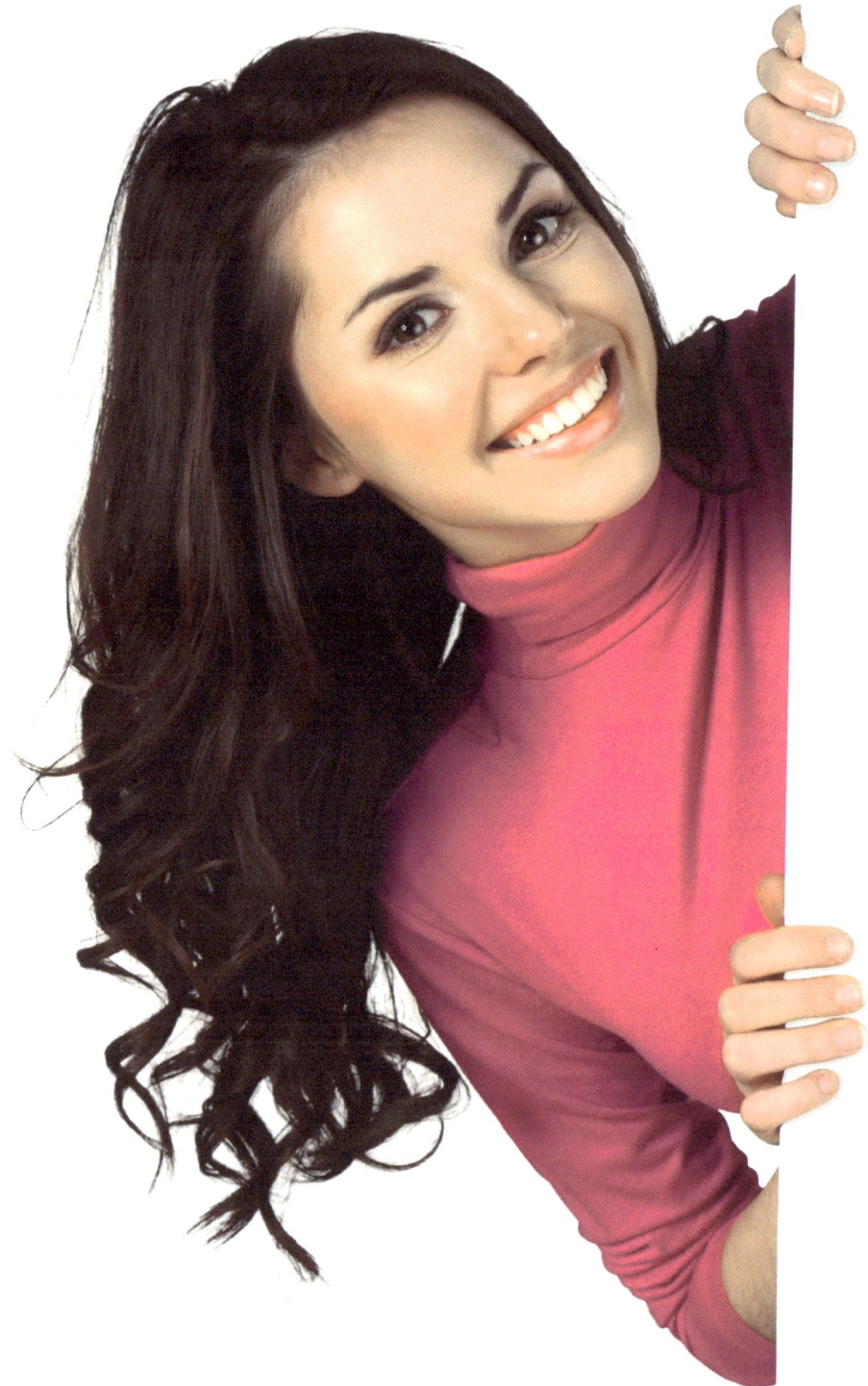

Day 32

Breathing through...

- I now understand that the world is within me.
- I can be at peace with myself.
- I can enjoy life.
- I am the master of my feelings.
- I can be protective of my boundaries.
- I believe in the Gifts within me.

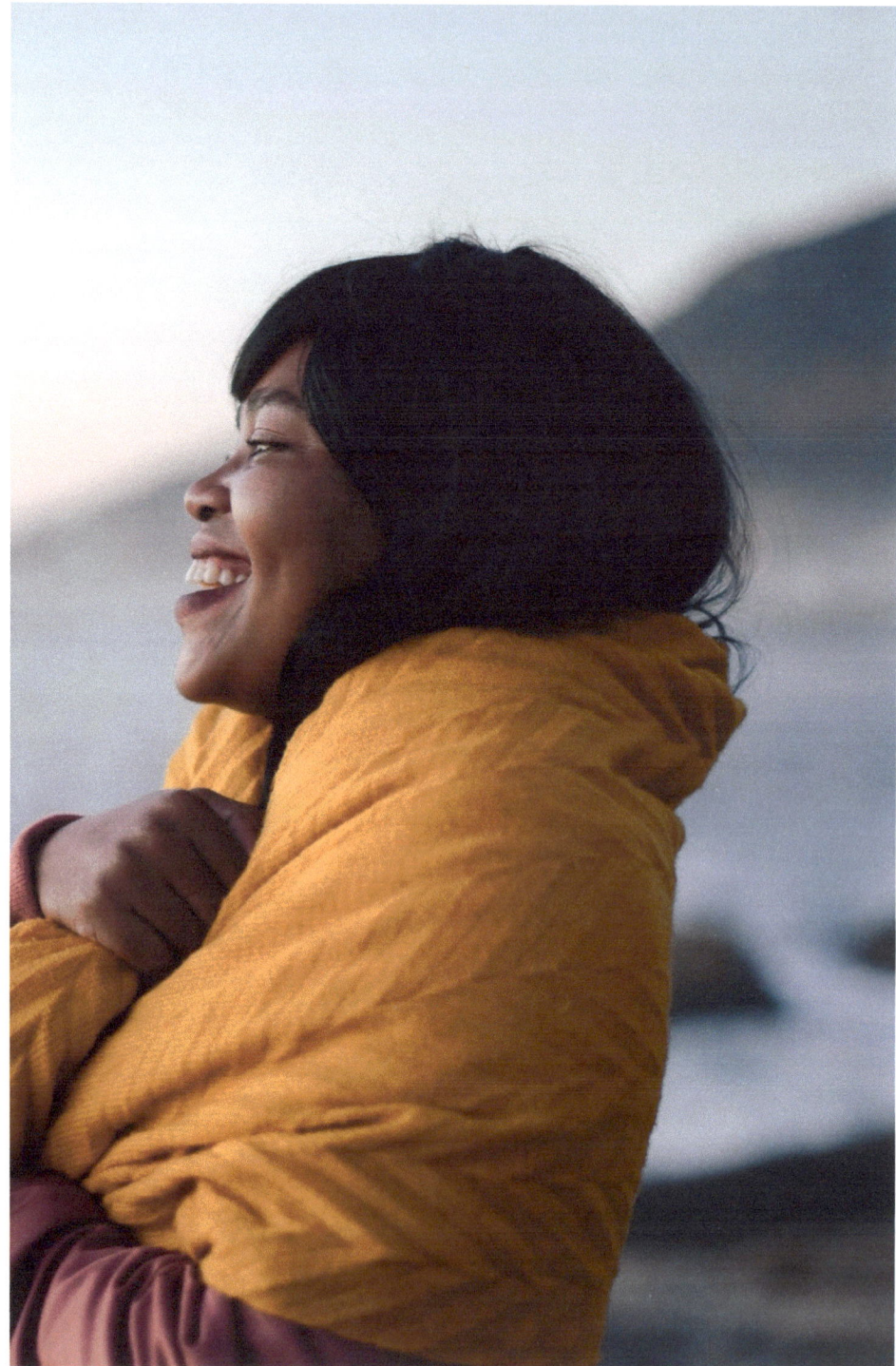

Day 33

Some meditate with their eyes
closed chanting a mantra, or eyes
open and being mindful.

I meditate with my eyes open
Because - All is Right here.
No words are necessary.
Being present with myself is rewarding
in itself As I am present with Me.
I feel complete and content Being Me.
I allow.

I now know more than ever -
I Matter - I HealWithin

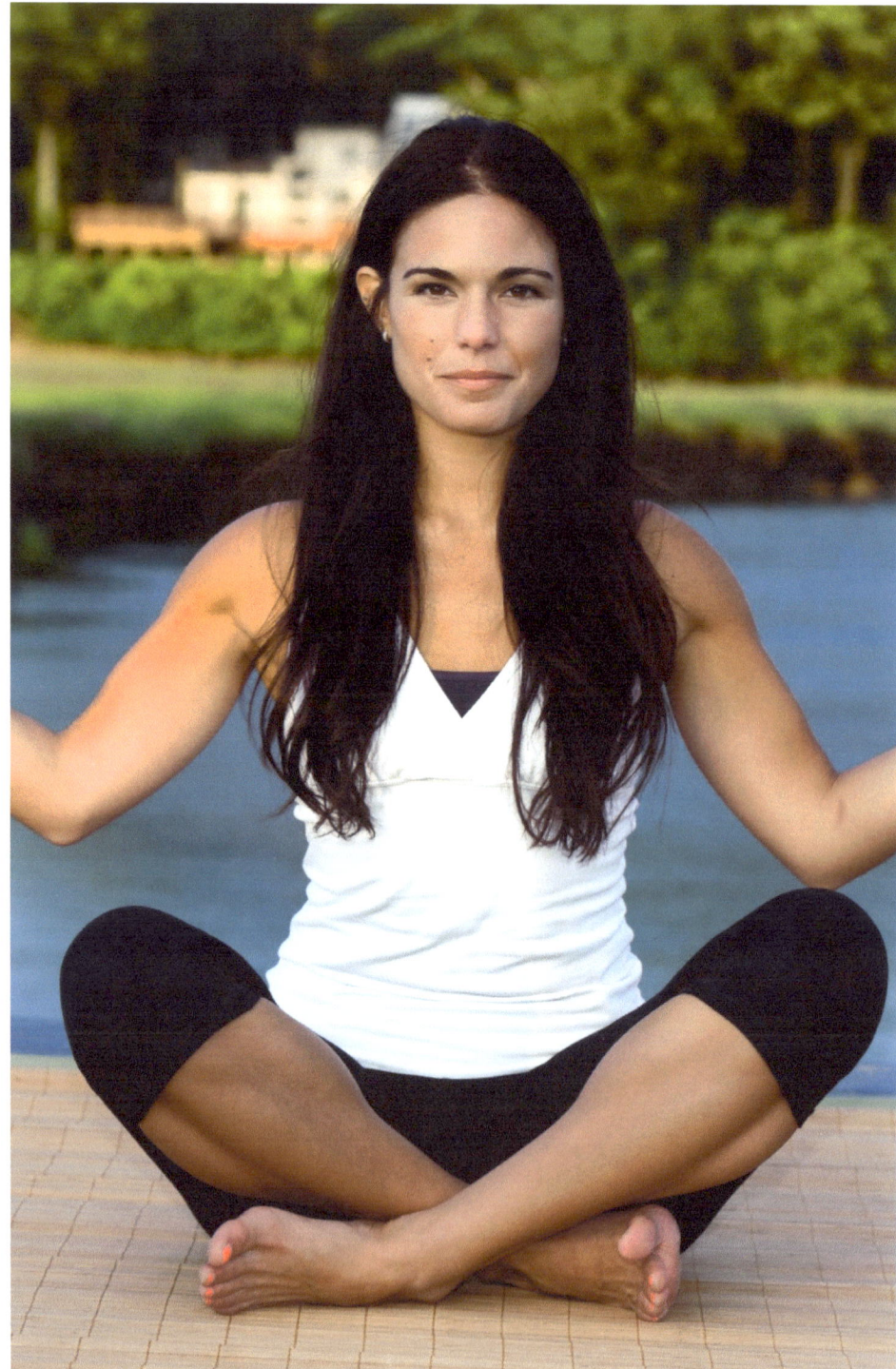

Daily Affirmations

1. I bring balance into my life for my mind, body, and soul.
2. I accept and appreciate myself far more deeply than ever before.
3. My body is strong and a safe place for me to be in.
4. I build trust every day.
5. My mind has a powerful healing effect on my body.
6. I am able to maintain my ideal weight.
7. I am highly motivated to exercise my body because I find exercise as fun.
8. I am aligned in my mind, body, and of my emotions.
9. I consciously create my own reality; everything in it is perfect.
10. I am safe in all my relationships; I am always treated well.
11. I trust the flow and process of life.
12. I'm happier with my body.
13. I am losing weight as I exercise.
14. I am perfectly healthy in body, mind, and spirit.
15. I nourish my mind, body, and soul.
16. I am grateful that my body tells me when something needs adjusting.
17. I am in control of my mind, body, spirit, and life.
18. I speak kindly to myself and about my body.
19. I trust myself with everything.

Daily Affirmations

20. I am losing weight as I eat right.
21. All the systems of my body function perfectly.
22. I learn from everything that happens in my life, and I trust my own intuition.
23. I am safe, supported, and protected at all times.
24. I now release all emotional and physical weight and burdens.
25. I am learning to trust my thought processes.
26. I love and approve of myself and my body.
27. Today, I put my full trust in my inner guidance.
28. Money is a state of consciousness. I allow prosperity to flow to me.
29. I release all negative energy from my body.
30. I let go and trust.
31. I have full confidence in myself.
32. I am safe and secure.
33. My body is listening to my loving self-talk.

Bonus Gift

Text "RELAX" to
818-221-2797
to download and
listen daily to
hypnosis audio
recording.

Narrated by Liza

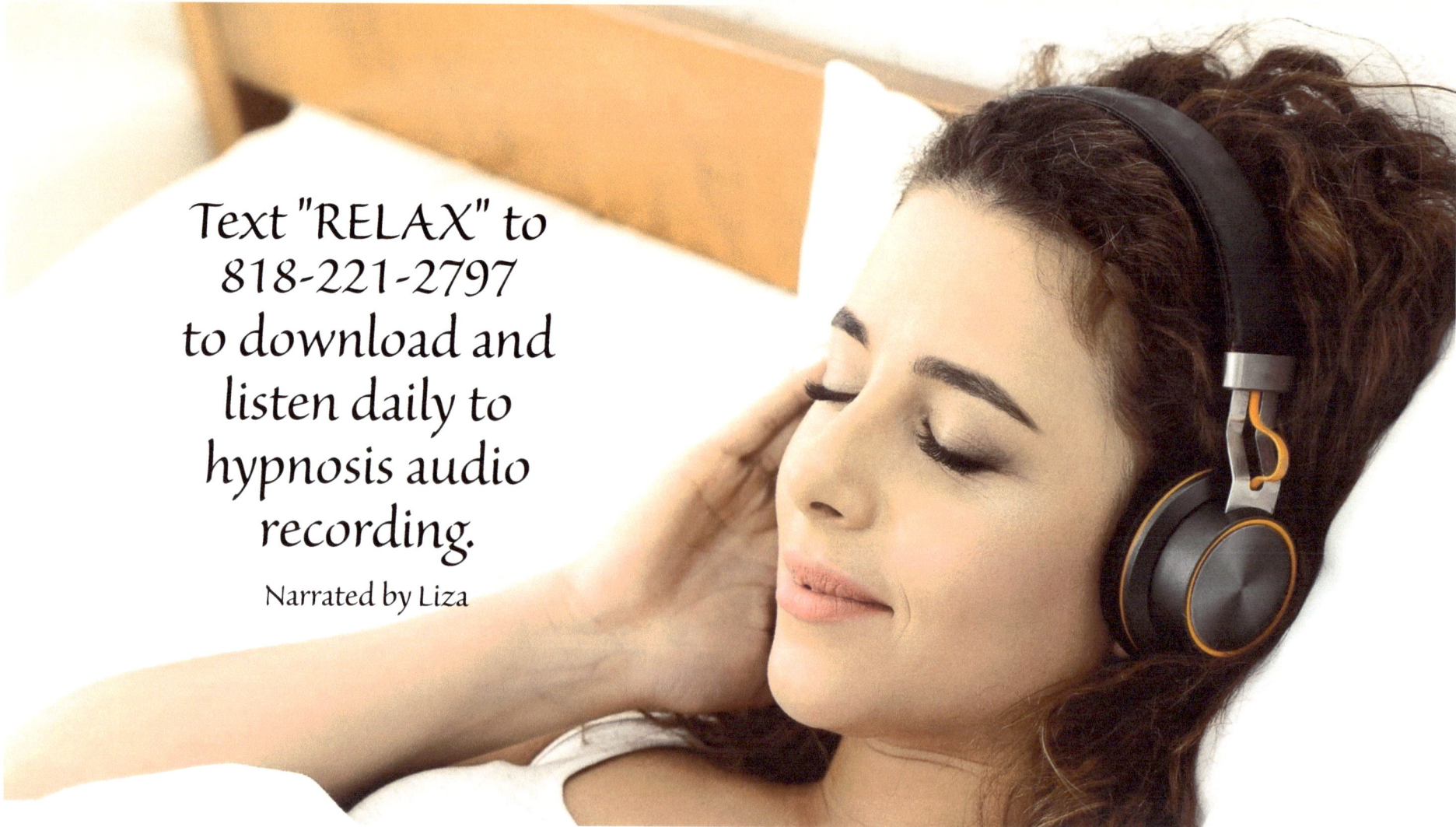

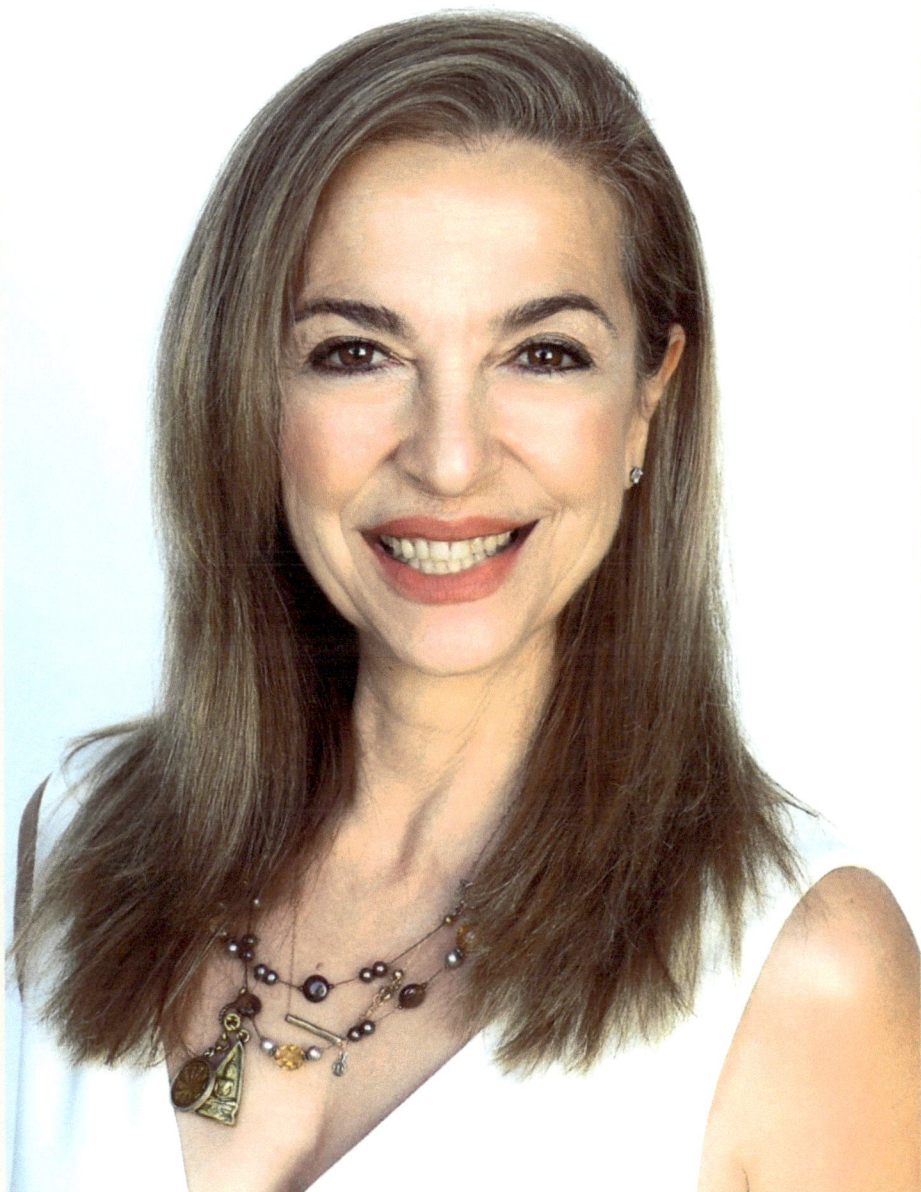

Liza Boubari

Founder of HealWithin

Enjoy the process as you...

Evoke past patterns
Embrace present reality
Evolve to desired SELF

Because "You Matter"

Liza takes you on a heartfelt journey of self-discovery and awareness through her 3E Method.

For more information or to work with Liza, text: I Matter to **818-221-2797**

www.ingramcontent.com/pod-product-compliance
Lightning Source LLC
Chambersburg PA
CBHW041553030426

42336CB00005B/61